About th

Liz Earle is a popular television ... author with a special interest in ... Prior to presenting her own series, *Beauty* ...-1, she spent 3 years as regular beauty presenter on ITV's *This Morning* programme. Her specialist knowledge and enthusiasm has made her reports compulsive viewing for millions nationwide. She is also a regular contributor to BBC and Independent radio.

An award-winning journalist, Liz has written for many national newspapers and magazines, and was formerly the health and beauty editor of *New Woman* magazine. She has a wealth of inside knowledge about the beauty business and is not afraid to explode many modern skincare myths. She also maintains a strong personal interest and belief in the importance of nutrition and complementary medicine.

For my parents:
thank you for giving me a skin
to save

SAVE YOUR SKIN

With Vital Oils

By the same author

VITAL OILS

SAVE YOUR SKIN
With Vital Oils

The Ultimate Anti-Ageing Plan for Smoother, Clearer Skin

LIZ EARLE

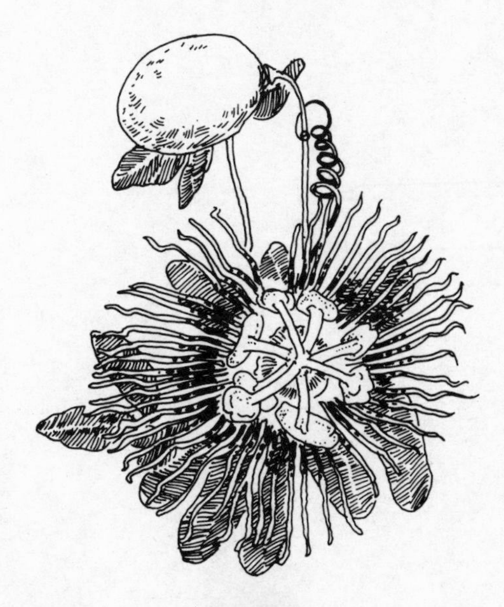

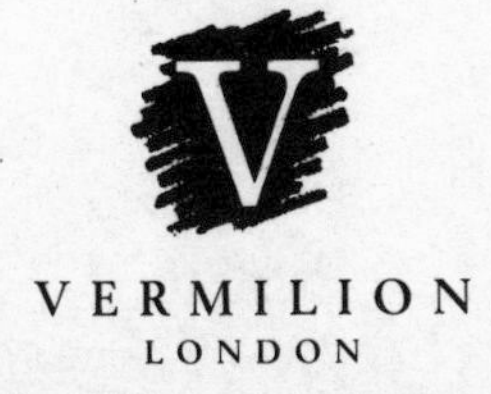

VERMILION
LONDON

Published in 1992 by Vermilion
an imprint of Ebury Press
Random Century House
20 Vauxhall Bridge Road
London SW1V 2SA

Catalogue record for this book is available from the British Library

ISBN 0 09 177172 2

Designed by: Bob Vickers
Illustrations by: Sue Sharples

Typeset in Palatino by Hope Services (Abingdon) Ltd
Printed in England by Mackays of Chatham Plc, Kent

Contents

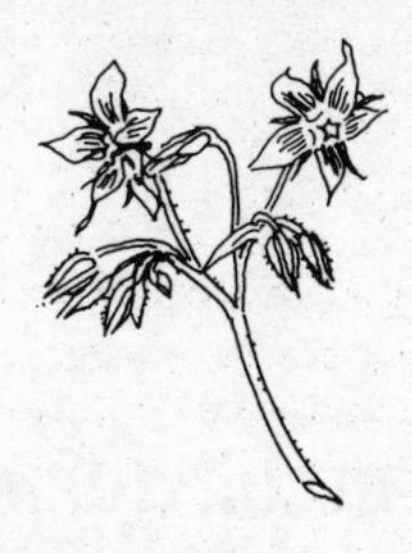

Acknowledgements

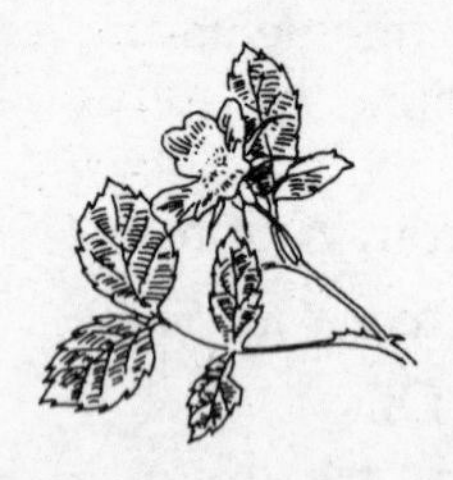

While writing this book, I have been lucky enough to work with some of the world's leading experts in both health and beauty. I should like to thank all those who freely gave me so much of their valuable time, especially Caroline Wheeler, Tom Hardman, Willem vas Dias, Val Holmes, Professor Albert Kligman, Dr John Hawk, Professor Ronald Marks, Dr David Ratsey, Amanda Ursell, Eve Lom, Patrick Holford and the Institute of Optimum Nutrition. I am grateful to the talented cookery writer, Eleanor Hale, for providing many of the deliciously inspired oil-enriched recipes; also to Beverly Benson, Sarah Collins and team, Rosie Sandberg and Claire Bowles. Last, but not least, my heartfelt thanks to Annie Bawtree for her patient re-typing; to Laura Hill for keeping Lily's tiny hands off my manuscript; and to Patrick for his support and (almost) unfailing sense of humour.

Introduction

At last, a simple, straightforward guide to looking after your skin. This unique plan provides foolproof advice on the successful treatment of spots and skin disorders. It also shows you how to delay the formation of fine lines, wrinkles and other visible signs of ageing. No expensive skin serum or magical elixir of youth works as well as this regime. All you need is the nutritional know-how to feed the skin from within and a simple, effective skincare programme.

British women spend a staggering £500 million every year on products promoted by the beauty industry for preventing the signs of ageing. However, not even the most expensive skin cream is able to penetrate the deeper layers of the skin or do more than surface repairs. Despite the millions spent, we continue to develop wrinkles and suffer from skin disorders and spots. While a moisturiser certainly makes the skin feel smoother, it cannot turn back the clock. However, there is a way to promote an eternally youthful glow and *Save Your Skin with Vital Oils* explains exactly how. One thing is certain – the only way to win the war on wrinkles is from within. Pure plant oils, such as passionflower oil and evening primrose oil, are powerful skin defenders. They contain the ingredients that reinforce every single skin cell, making them more resistant to the ageing process. Eating the right balance of natural oils prevents spots and pimples, smooths away skin rashes and keeps skin cells plump and strong. The result is a softer, firmer-looking face with greater elasticity and suppleness. Add this know-how to a natural skincare routine and you have the ultimate answer to beautiful skin.

Liz Earle

The Skin Savers

Three Simple Steps To Save Your Skin

1 Add a daily dose of vital oils to your diet
Vital oils are our best defence against ageing. Moisturisers and anti-ageing creams reach only dead surface skin cells, but the nutrients in plant oils are absorbed by the bloodstream and feed every living cell in the skin. This constant nourishment supplies our skin with the ingredients it needs to function effectively. It also strengthens the cellular membrane surrounding each cell, fights the destructive action of free-radicals (see page 00) and enzymes in the depths of the skin, and boosts the skins own natural moisture levels.

2 Always use a sunblock or sunscreen to save your skin from the sun
Your most valuable skincare product is a sunscreen to block out the sun's rays; shielding the skin from the extremely damaging radiation emitted by the sun is the most significant step in anti-ageing skincare. Even the relatively low levels of sunshine that reach our faces on a cloudy day can penetrate the skin and destroy its network of supporting elastin and collagen fibres. This is why the daily, routine use of a sunscreen is so important to preserve the face against premature ageing.

3 Work-out your face with regular exercise and massage
The muscles in your face need to be kept in good shape just as much as those in the rest of your body; a twice-weekly work-out of the muscles that support the skin prevents the facial tissues from becoming slack, and promotes stronger skin. A regular facial massage also brings much-needed oxygen supplies to the surface of the skin and speeds up the removal of the toxins that lead to spots and other skin disorders.

These three stages are the most important steps you will ever take towards saving your skin. Each is easy to do and, above all, highly effective. You will start to see an improvement immediately – and your face will thank you forever.

1

Beauty From Within

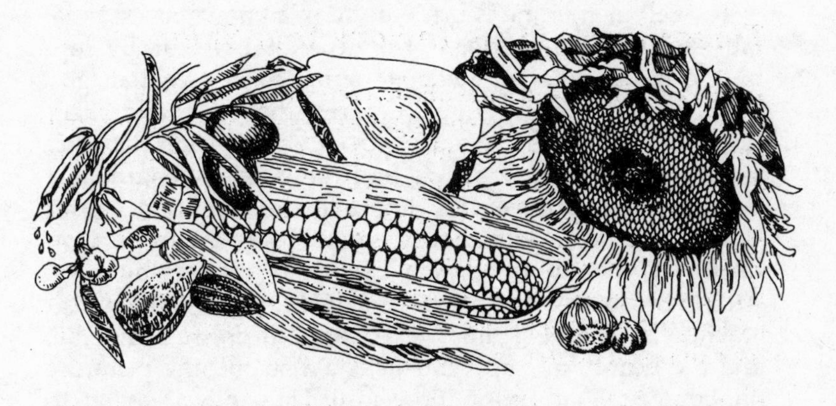

The food we eat has a major effect on the way our skin ages and behaves, because every single skin cell in the body relies on a constant supply of nutrients in order to flourish. Our skin cells suffer continual attacks from the environment and need a steady stream of nutritional defenders to help them win the war against wrinkles and other preventable skin disorders. The factors that cause the most damage to our skin are nutritional deficiencies, such as low vitamin levels; ultra-violet radiation from the sun; and poisonous pollutants, including car fumes and cigarette smoke. Fortunately for our skin, there are several ways we can minimise the damage that is done and keep our complexion in glowing good health. The most important starting point for stronger, smoother skin is a well-balanced diet that supplies the body with all the nutrients it requires to create a glowing complexion. Beauty comes from within, not out of a jar, and the only way to improve the way our faces look and feel is by fortifying our food with skin-strengthening nutrients.

If we feed our faces with the food it requires we can quickly improve the condition of our skin. Our skin is made up of millions of skin cells, each requiring specific amounts of nutrients in order to function healthily. The skin cells require good levels of vitamins and minerals, as well as many other nutrients that are a fundamental part of life. Each skin cell is surrounded by a protective coating called the cell membrane. This coating keeps the skin cell healthy and strong, and enables it to resist the destructive ageing processes which we will examine in detail a little later (see page 16).

The cell membrane is made up of oils known as essential fatty acids which we obtain from the food we eat. By supplying the body with adequate supplies of essential fatty acids we are effectively able to strengthen each and every skin cell membrane and achieve results far greater than any skin cream. So where do we find these skin-strengthening nutrients that dramatically improve the condition of our skin? The answer is that they are probably sitting in your kitchen cupboard or bathroom cabinet at this very moment. All vital plant oils are skin-savers, including unrefined vegetable oils, such as sunflower oil or cold-pressed olive oil, and the beauty oil supplements, such as evening primrose oil, borage oil and passionflower oil. These oils are 'vital' to a healthy skin, as well as to the whole body, because they contain three key elements that are needed to keep our complexions clear and youthful-looking. This trio of skin-treats comprises the three internal skin-savers:

- essential fatty acids (EFAs)
- natural vitamin E
- natural lecithin

Let us examine each of these three factors in closer detail to discover exactly how it is that they can save your skin.

Essential Fatty Acids

There is no doubt that fats in general have received a pretty bad press over the past few years, but is this really justified? The answer is a definite no, and both nutritionists and medics alike are increasingly coming to realise that some fats are very important for the health of our skin as well as for our overall health. The fundamental point about oils and fats is to know exactly which ones the body needs to survive and, perhaps more importantly, which ones should be avoided. My earlier book on this subject, *Vital Oils* (Vermilion, 1991) was the first to link the value of oils directly to improving the way we look and feel. *Vital Oils* contains a two-week oil-enriched diet plan (yes, you do lose weight provided you know which type of oils to use and which fats to avoid). Those who followed the diet reported quite remarkable results from simply adding a small amount of pure, natural plant oil to their diet every day. The diet quickly became known as the Vital Oils Beauty Diet because it made such a dramatic difference to the appearance.

The benefits of adding oils to the diet include:

- clearer skin
- a softer and less-lined complexion
- shinier, more manageable hair
- stronger, longer nails

In addition to improving the way we look, these vital oils bring many health benefits. Those who followed the oil-enriched eating plan experienced better health; the most common improvements were as follows:

- fewer symptoms of inflammatory disorders, such as arthritis
- reduced cholesterol levels and therefore less risk of heart disease
- fewer allergy disorders
- fewer signs of stress
- relief from Pre-Menstrual Syndrome

These results clearly illustrate the facts that have been known throughout the medical world for some time: the ingredients in oils are essential both for good health and glowing good looks.

Eating the wrong type of fats

In the affluent Western world of the 1990s there is no doubt that we all eat far too much of the wrong type of fat. The World Health Organisation has stated that saturated animal fats (see Glossary) are a significant health risk in Western European countries, and the British government has set new guidelines that urge us to cut our fat consumption drastically.

Fats in the diet have been subject to an enormous number of studies in many different countries, and the fact that eating the wrong type of fat is dangerous to our health is accepted by all the major health organisations worldwide.

Canadian fat expert, Udo Erasmus, illustrated the potency of a high-fat diet by stating that diseases of fatty degeneration kill upwards of 75 per cent of the people living in the affluent, industrialised nations in the 1990s. This indicates just how critical it is to maintain the right balance of oil and fat in our diet. However, not all fats are bad for us and some are needed for many bodily functions, including strong, supple skin.

Spot the difference

All oils and fats have a similar chemical composition, but fats tend to be solid at room temperature whereas oils are always liquid. Both are made up of fatty acids which are the major building blocks of the fats in the human body. In addition to being an important source of energy, fatty acids are the largest structural component of the membrane that surrounds each cell in the body. They also have a special function in helping to build and maintain healthy cells, so they are needed at the very beginning of life and are important to continuing good health within the body. Fatty acids also form the fat that surrounds our internal organs, providing insulation and shock absorption. They have additional roles in areas of active tissue functioning, such as the brain and sense organs, and are needed to create the biological regulators called prostaglandins.

A severe shortage of fatty acids can be fatal, and even a mild deficiency can quickly cause the skin to become dry and leathery and to age far more quickly. Those who embark on a fat-free weight-loss diet soon notice that their complexion becomes dull and dehydrated, their hair lacks lustre and their nails become brittle. This is because certain fats and oils contain ingredients that work as *internal moisturisers* and the key to developing a stronger, clearer skin lies in knowing which oils and fats to use and which to avoid. Our consumption of animal fats should certainly be minimised or avoided altogether, while eating the right sorts of fats is absolutely essential. The difference between 'good' and 'bad' fats is straightforward as they can be split neatly into two groups: fats tend to be made up of saturated fatty acids and are 'bad' for us, whereas oils almost always consist of monounsaturated or polyunsaturated fatty acids and are 'good' for us. The difference between the two groups of animal fats and vegetable oils is not only important for good health, but is fundamental to a good complexion.

saturates (animal fat)	*monounsaturates* (vegetable oil)	*polyunsaturates* (vegetable oil)
lard	olive oil	safflower oil
dripping	almond oil	sunflower oil
suet	sesame oil	corn (maize) oil
milk		
cream	hazelnut oil	walnut oil
butter		rapeseed oil
cheese		soybean oil
egg yolk		peanut (groundnut) oil

Saturated fats

These fats are easy to spot as they are solid at room temperature. Examples of saturated fats are butter, dripping, suet, lard, fatty meat and hard margarine. All saturated fats contain potentially harmful saturated fatty acids and, in most cases, large amounts of cholesterol. We know that eating too many of these substances is the major cause of coronary heart disease and other degenerative disorders, such as cancer of the colon and breast. Saturated fats block the arteries and slow down the removal of waste matter and toxins by clogging up our lymphatic system. This results in a build-up of debris in the lower levels of the skin, leading to spots, pimples and a sallow-looking complexion. Unfortunately, many modern foods are full of saturated fats – look at the labels on the packaged foods in your fridge and see how many of them contain saturated fats. However, there are some simple steps we can take to help cut down our intake of saturated fats:

- eat less meat and always trim off any visible fat
- switch to lower-fat meats, such as chicken, turkey and game
- eat more fish and seafood
- choose extra-lean mince for cooking

- grill, bake or poach foods instead of frying them
- switch from full-fat to skimmed or semi-skimmed milk
- replace cream with low-fat yoghurt or low-fat fromage frais
- avoid foods which contain 'invisible' saturated fats, such as cakes, biscuits, pastries, ice-cream and crisps

Monounsaturated and polyunsaturated fats
These are the good guys of the fat world. Monounsaturated fats, such as olive oil, are liquid at room temperature but begin to solidify if kept in the fridge. Polyunsaturated fats, such as vegetable and fish oils, are liquid at room temperature and below. Polyunsaturated fats contain essential fatty acids which, as their name suggests, are absolutely *essential* for health; without them the body would disintegrate. Although the body can make its own supplies of monounsaturates it cannot produce polyunsaturates so all our supplies must come from the foods that we eat. We only need a small amount of essential fatty acids, but we must make sure the body receives its quota every single day.

Essential fatty acids are used to build the fragile membrane that surrounds every cell in the body. By reinforcing the membranes surrounding the skin cells, essential fatty acids also prevent water loss and keep skin cells healthy and strong. However, the essential fatty acids in these cellular membranes are destroyed by fat-soluble substances, such as alcohol, barbiturates, many prescription drugs and carcinogenic chemicals. Essential fatty acids are also needed to preserve the protective lipidic barrier that sits between the upper and lower levels of the skin to prevent moisture evaporation. This is why adding a daily dose of vital oils to your diet makes such a visible difference to your skin's texture and appearance. In the longer term, these essential fatty acids encourage the replacement of stronger collagen and elastin fibres in the dermis and so help to prevent the skin sagging and wrinkling.

The case against hydrogenation

The most common monounsaturated oils are olive oil and sesame oil, while those richest in polyunsaturates include sunflower, safflower, corn, rapeseed and soybean oil. Both types will help prevent heart disease by unclogging the arteries and preventing a build-up of fatty deposits that lead to arteriosclerosis (hardening of the arteries). However, polyunsaturates should only be eaten in their natural form as liquid vegetable oils. When they are hardened, or *hydrogenated* (combined with hydrogen), to turn them into solid fats for making hard margarine, low-fat spreads and processed foods, their chemical structure changes and they behave like saturated fats in the body. It is worth noting that in the one study that has claimed low-fat diets have no effect on heart disease, the testers were fed on foods high in hydrogenated fats. It is not surprising, therefore, that their results were so poor. Perhaps more worryingly, hardened or hydrogenated vegetable oils convert the healthy 'cis' fatty acids into unhealthy 'trans' fatty acids (see Glossary) which should be avoided.

Not all brands of margarine or low-fat spread contain hydrogenated fats and it is worth seeking out the healthier versions in health food shops. These should clearly state that they are made with unhydrogenated vegetable oils or that they contain high levels of the 'cis' form of fatty acids (read the small print on the label). Basically, the best way to ruin the nutritional value of a perfectly healthy plant oil is to hydrogenate it. Had hydrogenation been a recent discovery by food processors, it probably would have been banned, says Herbert Dutton, one of the most knowledgeable and renowned oil chemists in North America. He states that because of all the known and unknown effects on health and the "complexity of isomers formed during hydrogenation", government regulations passed to protect our health would forbid its use in any edible products. As it is, hydrogenation has been used since the 1930s on a frighteningly large scale and now has a powerful industry behind it. (Check the ingredients on the foods in your kitchen to see just how prevalent the process is.)

Apart from the risk of hydrogenation, another potential problem with polyunsaturated oils is that they break down rapidly at high temperatures to produce damaging peroxides, so they should not be used for frying. Sunflower and safflower oils, for example, are wonderfully healthy oils but should be kept for using cold in salad dressing or mayonnaise. Monounsaturated oils, such as olive oil, are much more stable and are better for recipes that require heating. All oils, notably polyunsaturated oils, start to go rancid by oxidising with the air immediately after opening. Do not leave the bottle open for longer than necessary and protect the oil from light and heat. Light speeds up the reaction of the oil with oxygen by one thousand times; standing a bottle of oil in a sunny corner of the kitchen is one of the fastest ways to turn it rancid. All vegetable oils are best bought in small quantities that can be finished quickly and kept in a cool, dark place, such as in the fridge.

The Vital Oils connection

Unrefined vegetable oils and natural fish oils contain many of the nutrients needed to encourage better-looking skin. The two main polyunsaturated fatty acids which the body *must* obtain through food are linoleic acid and alpha linoleic acid. Other important substances found in unrefined plant oils include natural Vitamin E and small amounts of lecithin, and we shall examine the skin-saving properties of each of these substances later in this chapter. However, the key word to look for when choosing any cooking oil is 'unrefined'. This guarantees that the valuable nutrients we need have not been removed during the oil's processing. Unfortunately, most vegetable oils found on the supermarket shelves are heavily refined, bland, lifeless and devoid of nutrients. Cold-pressed oils such as olive oil are usually unrefined but watch out for the confusingly labelled 'pure' olive oil which has been processed. Other unrefined oils, including sunflower, safflower, sesame, walnut, hazelnut and corn oils can be found in good health food shops.

Omega-6 essential fatty acids

There are two main groups of essential fatty acids that affect the skin. The first is known as the Omega-6 series and those with a working knowledge of chemistry will recognise that they have been given this name because their chemical structure includes a double link between the sixth and seventh carbon atoms. The Omega-6 group of essential fatty acids comes from linoleic acid which is found in most vegetable oils, nuts, seeds and leafy vegetables. You might think that lettuce is fat-free but even this slimmers' friend contains tiny amounts of linoleic acid. This essential fatty acid is especially important for the skin as it is used as the inter-cellular cement that holds skin cells together in the epidermis. If our diet is deficient in linoleic acid, gaps appear within the cells, causing moisture loss and skin dehydration, and eventually eczema-like skin eruptions, hair loss, dry skin, drying up of glands, arthritis, and heart and circulatory problems. Linoleic acid is the essential fatty acid that is most needed by the body as it is required by every living cell, as well as by the immune system, and a prolonged absence of linoleic acid from the diet is fatal. When absorbed by the body, linoleic acid is broken down into smaller components, the most well known being gamma linolenic acid (GLA).

Linoleic acid into GLA

The Omega-6 group of essential fatty acids comes from the parent linoleic acid found in nuts, seeds, leafy vegetables and plant oils. In an ideal world, we absorb the natural linoleic acid found in these foods and the body converts it into other essential fatty acids such as GLA. This particular essential fatty acid has been found to have potent skincare properties and can heal many kinds of skin disorders, ranging from acne to eczema. Although the body has the ability to convert the linoleic acid into GLA, this process frequently breaks down. Factors that interfere with its conversion include most of the hazards of modern living, including:

- stress
- pollution
- viral infections
- alcohol
- saturated fats
- many medications

Unless you lead a blameless lifestyle, it may be advisable to ensure your supplies of GLA are kept high by taking an oil supplement which contains this fatty acid in a pre-digested form.

GLA for baby-soft skin

Ready-made GLA is rare, but can be obtained from a few

sources, such as borage oil and evening primrose oil, which is why these oils are often added to nutritional supplements. GLA is especially important for infants and is found in human breast milk, although it is not added to formula milks in Britain. Long-term studies reported in *The Lancet* medical journal have linked the fats found in breast milk to brain development. It has been established that premature babies given their mother's milk by tube had, by the time they reached the age of seven or eight, significantly higher IQs than those who were fed on formula milk.

Another more immediate side-effect for many babies fed only on formula milk is chronically dry skin or atopic eczema due to lack of GLA in the diet. Studies have shown that children who develop this type of eczema have unusually low levels of essential fatty acids in their blood. The simplest and safest way to treat the symptoms of atopic eczema or dry skin in babies is to add a few drops of borage oil or evening primrose oil to each formula feed. This is something I did under paediatric guidance for my own daughter when I stopped breastfeeding, and it significantly improved the softness and condition of her skin. Although the formula feed manufacturers have decided not to add GLA to British powdered milks (because, I am told, it would shorten their shelf-life), the Japanese consider it important enough to import British-grown evening primrose oil for this very purpose.

High levels of GLA in the bloodstream, whether converted from linoleic acid from fresh foods or taken directly in the form of oil supplement capsules, plays an important part in protecting our skin from within. GLA has been found to strengthen skin cells, increase their moisture content and regulate severe skin disorders. GLA is also needed to create and act on the prostaglandins that are involved with almost every procedure in the body. By controlling our prostaglandins, GLA can improve many hormone-related disorders, such as Pre-Menstrual Syndrome and symptoms of the menopause. This is one reason why evening primrose oil supplements are now taken by so many women worldwide. GLA also improves the action of the T-lymphocytes that engulf foreign particles and remove them from the system. This leads to a clearer complexion, encourages skin healing and promotes healthy scar tissue.

Omega-3 EFAs and the Eskimos

The second group of essential fatty acids important for a healthy skin is the Omega-3 series which are found mainly in fish oils. Those interested in the technicalities may like to know that they are called the Omega-3 series because of the double link between the third and fourth carbon atoms in their chemical structure. The first clues that fish oils could dramatically improve our health came when Eskimos, who eat a diet based largely on whale blubber, fatty fish and seal meat, were found to have no incidence of heart disease or diabetes. This was despite the fact that their diet contained a high proportion of animal fats. It was discovered that the oils in fatty fish are a rich source of Omega-3 essential fatty acids and these protect us from many disorders, including heart disease. Fish oils contain two ingredients that have been found to reduce significantly the risk of coronary heart disease and strokes. These are eicosapentaenoic acid (EPA), which is converted into prostaglandins, and docosahexaenoic acid (DHA), which regulates their activity. The only places where DHA can be found in land animals is in the brain, eyeball, adrenal glands and testicles. This probably explains why so many cultures have traditionally considered these parts of the body to be rare delicacies and dishes of sheep's eyeballs and monkey brains may still be served to honoured guests in the Far East today. Due to the fact that DHA deteriorates rapidly, these tasty morsels must be eaten from a very freshly slaughtered animal, which only goes to show that a spoonful of cod liver oil is really quite an attractive proposition after all!

Fish oils and heart disease

Taking fish oil supplements and eating more fatty fish, such as mackerel and herring, have become accepted as mainstream medical factors for controlling the occurrence of coronary heart disease. A blend of fish oils in capsules is even available on prescription for those with dangerously high blood fat levels.

Fish oils and asthma

Studies carried out in France in 1991 indicate that supplements of fish oils containing EPA and DHA may also help some sufferers of asthma. The pulmonary function of asthma patients was monitored during a double-blind clinical trial and, although no immediate benefits were noticed, there were definite longer-term improvements. The forced expiratory volume (FEV) of those taking a daily dose of 1g of fish oils was reported as increasing by 23 per cent after a period of 9 months. It is well known that fish oil fatty acids modify the metabolism of prostaglandins and pro-inflammatory cytokines that lead to swelling, so there is a strong theoretical basis that they help cases of asthma linked to chronic inflammation.

Fish oils and arthritis

Not only do the essential fatty acids in fish oils regulate blood fats within the body but they also modulate the types of prostaglandins that control inflammation. This is one reason why cod liver oil and other fish oils work so well as an anti-inflammatory treatment for painful arthritis and rheumatism.

Fish oils and skin disorders

The essential fatty acids EPA and DHA are also able to target the inflammatory leukotrienes that are found in abnormally high levels amongst eczema and psoriasis sufferers, and can lead to lower levels being produced. Although no claims are made that cod liver oil or fish oils can cure these skin disorders, they certainly seem to help many sufferers who take them regularly over a period of time. EPA and DHA are also important components of the membranes surrounding all our cells, including skin cells, and can help keep the complexion supple and strong.

Vitamin E

Vitamin E was discovered in 1922 when researchers noticed that something in lettuce prevented sterility in animals that had been fed on rancid fats. The unknown substance was called vitamin E as it directly followed the discovery of vitamins A, B, C and D. It was also termed 'tocopherol' because it promoted healthy offspring; the word was derived from the Greek *tokos*, meaning childbirth, and *phero*, meaning to bring forth. Since those early years, our knowledge about the importance of vitamin E has grown rapidly and in 1968 it was officially recognised as an 'essential' vitamin. This means that the body cannot function properly without it and that all supplies must come from our diet.

Vitamin E is a fat-soluble vitamin so it only dissolves in oils (such as vegetable oils), fats and alcohol. In order for it to be used by the body it must first be emulsified by bile salts secreted from the liver. The vitamin is dispersed into tiny droplets which are then absorbed into the bloodstream and the lymphatic system. From here the nutrient is distributed throughout the body and any leftover reserves are stored away in adipose (fat) tissues, the liver and muscles for future use.

The free radical connection

Vitamin E is an anti-oxidant and, as such, prevents damage due to by-products of oxidation in the body. Oxidation itself is a chemical reaction that provides our cells with energy and is essential for life. However, if the process of oxidation gets out of hand it may generate damaging free radicals. These highly destructive particles come from two sources, internal and external.

Internal free radicals are produced continually by the body due to unrestrained releases of oxygen, and have limited benefits in combating bacteria. If allowed to get out of control, however, free radicals quickly multiply and set about destroying cells and damaging vital cellular material, including the deoxyribonucleic acid (DNA) that creates life itself. When a free radical attacks a cell it combines with the important polyunsaturated (or essential) fatty acids in the cell membrane to produce lipid peroxides. These in turn generate more free radicals, creating a chain-reaction of destruction.

External sources of free radicals are a growing problem for the skin as well as the health of the whole body. They include the following:

- nitrogen dioxide and ozone in polluted air
- heavy metals such as lead and mercury
- ionizing radiation and strong sunshine
- car exhaust fumes

- cigarette smoke
- pesticides
- organic solvents
- food additives
- food irradiation

Rancid fats and oils also increase our levels of free radicals and their toxic peroxides. All told, modern living has dramatically increased our exposure to these damaging elements and we are ever more at risk of their ill-effects. Free radicals cause premature skin ageing and are believed to play a significant part in cancer, cataracts and many other degenerative diseases. These potent particles also inactivate enzymes and proteins, cause mutations that lead to cancer and alter our cells' response to hormones and neurotransmitters, the chemical substances released from nerve endings that transmit messages between the nerves and the muscles or glands that they are connected to.

The ageing factor

The buzz-words in modern skincare are 'free radical fighter' as these destructive particles are acknowledged to be the major ageing factor within the skin. Free-radicals specifically destroy collagen and elastin fibres and reduce the rate of cell renewal. Vitamin E is vitally important because it acts as a free radical scavenger, mopping up these destructive particles and neutralising their harmful effects. This valiant vitamin also reduces the lipidic peroxidation that damages the skin cells' essential fatty acids as we age.

In addition to fighting free radicals, vitamin E also acts on other toxic particles called nitrosamines, which are known cancer-causing agents. Nitrosamines are produced when frying certain foods, such as bacon, and vitamin E had been reported to reduce their harmful effect dramatically. A simple way to put this knowledge to good use is to fry your rashers in unrefined vegetable oils which have retained their natural vitamin E content. However, most recent data suggests that considerably more vitamin E than is currently eaten in the average diet is necessary to prevent all free radical cell damage.

So important is the role of anti-oxidant nutrients, such as vitamin E, that in 1991 the British government gave £1.65 million to fund a research project into the study of their activities. Vitamin E is one of the few substances (along with fish oils) that defends the body against an inflammatory group of chemicals called leukotrienes which have been implicated in rheumatoid arthritis, eczema and psoriasis.

Vitamin E and the skin

Vitamin E is also known to heal the skin, and it has many other useful skincare properties. Studies have revealed that natural vitamin E can help several severe skin disorders and works well on all skin types. In cases of chronically dry and dehydrated complexions, vitamin E increases the amount of moisture retained within the skin to help prevent dryness and flaking. Vitamin E molecules are tiny, so they are able to penetrate the skin; in fact, it is one of the few cosmetic ingredients genuinely able to slip through the skin to moisturise from within.

Experiments show that vitamin E is absorbed in two ways. Firstly, it passes through the upper-epidermis into the intermediary basal layer and down into the lower dermis. It can also slip through the pilo-sebaceous glands and the interior of hair follicles (but not through the sweat ducts). Studies show that within 6–24 hours of application, significant amounts of vitamin E can be found in the fine capillaries of the lower dermis. When applied topically, the vitamin seems to head more for the smallest capillary than when taken internally and distributed via the bloodstream and lymphatic system. This suggests that applying vitamin E directly to the surface of the skin is an important part of vitamin E therapy. Similarly, a few hours after applying vitamin E directly to the hair, traces of the nutrient can be found in the central cortex of each hair strand.

Face preserver

In addition to its moisturising and anti-free radical properties, vitamin E is also a natural preservative and is included in many facial moisturisers to prevent them from becoming rancid once opened. The nutrient is also added to some hand creams as it has been found to counteract irritation and reduce the damaging potential of all household detergents, such as washing-up liquid. It also has therapeutic uses and vitamin E ointment applied to the skin has been found to help some patients suffering from eczema and psoriasis. While it is good for dry skin conditions, vitamin E can also be used on oily skins and can even help heal acne. This is because it reduces sebum production in the skin and prevents the formation of milia (whiteheads). Research carried out by the Henkel Corporation in Illinois has shown that sebum production can be reduced by as much as 73 per cent, and that vitamin E is effective in acne treatment both by reducing sebum levels and by suppressing the inflammation caused by oxidative processes within the skin.

Burns, scars and scalds also respond well to topical treatment with vitamin E. Severe facial injuries, such as those inflicted by being thrown through a windscreen in a car crash, have been helped with daily applications of vitamin E ointment. Vitamin E has the power to regenerate and repair damaged skin tissues so it is increasingly used in hospital burns units and in intensive care. Large doses of vitamin E have been found to speed up the healing process quite dramatically, as well as to fade scar tissue rapidly. Even long established scars and stretch marks can be faded by taking 500 iu of vitamin E every day and rubbing the contents of a capsule directly into the affected area. Vitamin E also works well in this way to treat sunburn and scalding, and it is worth keeping a small bottle of wheatgerm oil in the first aid box for this purpose. The high concentration of vitamin E in wheatgerm oil can result in temporary flushing or reddening of the skin as fresh blood supplies are brought to the surface, but this is not harmful and proves that the vitamin has a very real action. Some types of synthetic vitamin E have been known to cause skin irritation and allergic reactions when used on the face, so it is safer to stick to the natural version found in wheatgerm and other plant oils.

Vitamin E for a healthy heart

Besides being one of our great skin defenders, vitamin E is an outstanding nutrient in many other ways. Studies show that vitamin E reduces the amount of oxygen our cells, muscles and organs need to function. This is tremendous news as it enables more oxygen to be utilised within the body. Doctors treating heart disease with high doses of vitamin E in Canada photographed the hearts of patients suffering from a decreased blood supply. After vitamin E therapy, the new set of photographs clearly showed areas of regeneration as a result of oxygen conservation. This ability to restore life to previously decaying areas of the body has earned vitamin E the nickname 'vitality vitamin'. The regenerative powers of vitamin E are also of benefit to the skin as they enable skin cells to function as effectively on less oxygen, releasing supplies to oxygen-starved cells that would otherwise die.

This versatile nutrient is also needed to increase muscle tone and strength, to regulate blood clotting to reduce the risk of thrombosis and to even out the complexion by preventing patches of discolouration beneath the surface of the skin. Vitamin E is particularly important in the dermis as it strengthens the tiny capillary walls and encourages the larger blood vessels to dilate or widen. This reduces blood pressure and allows an increased flow of blood to deliver more oxygen to the cells, at the same time carrying away additional waste matter.

The risk of deficiency

Despite its obvious importance, many of us risk a vitamin E deficiency due to its systematic removal from our diet. The refining of wheat, the loss of vitamins in food during refining processes, food additives and the pollution of soil in which our food is grown have all conspired to deplete our vitamin E levels greatly. The richest source of vitamin E is pure wheatgerm, or wheatgerm oil, which contains 190 mg per 100 g. If we take the production of white bread as an example, we see that the wheatgerm that contains 90 per cent of the plant's vitamins and minerals is removed from the grain before grinding. After the flour has been ground it is bleached white and this removes the remaining 10 per cent of its vitamins. From nature's richest natural source of this valuable nutrient, we end up with a food product that contains virtually no vitamin E at all.

Vegetable oils, such as safflower oil, corn oil and soybean oil are also excellent sources of vitamin E. After refining, bleaching and deodorising, however, they lose almost their entire vitamin quota. This illustrates why it is so important to buy pure, unrefined or cold-pressed cooking oils that still retain their vitamin E. The label on a bottle of oil usually states whether the oil is unrefined; if in any doubt, choose the darkest coloured and strongest smelling oil as this usually indicates a minimum of processing. Vitamin E neutralises the free radicals and toxic peroxides that cause oils to turn rancid, so unrefined oils containing vitamin E will keep far longer once opened.

The vitamin E naturally present in unrefined vegetable oils is also there for another reason. Although the polyunsaturated fatty acids in oils, such as sunflower and safflower oil, are beneficial to the body, they require the presence of vitamin E to stabilise and protect them. If we increase our intake of these fatty acids without balancing them with adequate levels of vitamin E, the body must release the vitamin E that it has stored in the liver. Eventually, the liver runs out of its reserves and we become deficient in one of our most important nutrients.

The damage done to skin cells and to the rest of the body by a vitamin E deficiency occurs slowly over decades. Unlike other vitamins, there are no immediate signs that the body lacks this important nutrient. Usually the first signs that we are vitamin E deficient are premature ageing of the skin, wrinkles and muscle wastage, but by then it is too late to reverse the damage. Protecting the state of our skin and our internal health must be part of a long-term strategy and you are never too old – or too young – to start. The answer is simply to take a daily dose of vitamin E in the form of a supplement, such as wheatgerm oil, or in a beauty oil supplement that is enriched with natural vitamin E, or by cooking with the right type of vegetable oils (see chart). When choosing supplements, however, it must be said that the natural vitamin E extracted from wheatgerm is far more effective than its synthetic counterpart which is produced as a petrochemical by-product. Officially, natural vitamin E is 36 per cent more potent than the synthetic type, but recent studies suggest that it is more likely to be twice as effective. The type of vitamin E in your multi-vitamins should be stated on the label, albeit in tiny print. Natural vitamin E is listed as d-alpha-tocopherol, while the synthetic version is dl-alpha-tocopherol. Alternatively, vitamin supplements containing natural vitamin E sometimes state that it is from a 100 per cent natural source.

Vitamin E levels in unrefined oils

Per 100 g	*approximate units of Vitamin E*
Wheatgerm oil	175
Sunflower oil	72
Safflower oil	59
Peanut (groundnut) oil	28
Cod liver oil	20
Soybean oil	12
Avocado oil	2

Other useful sources of natural vitamin E are raw sunflower seeds, almonds, eggs and whole grains. Wholemeal bread also provides the body with a good supply and contains nearly 10 times more vitamin E than white bread.

Lecithin

In addition to the vitamins, there is another skin-saving nutrient found in plant oils called lecithin (pronounced less-e-thin). This yellowish-brown substance is named from the Greek for egg yolk, where it was first isolated. Although lecithin is neither a vitamin nor a mineral, it contains both types of nutrients, plus the essential fatty acid linoleic acid. While often overlooked by both the nutritional and medical world, lecithin plays an important part in all living beings, from humans to animals and even plants. Lecithin occurs naturally in the membrane surrounding all living cells and, in humans, the highest concentrations can be found in the brain, liver, kidneys and bone marrow.

Lecithin is also one of the many substances that make up a cocktail of compounds called Natural Moisturising Factors (NMFs) found in the skin. Natural Moisturising Factors include hyaluronic acid, urea, lactic acid, mucopolysaccharides and phospholipids such as lecithin. These agents are all powerful internal moisturisers and work by absorbing moisture from the atmosphere and holding on to it within the skin. They can also be made synthetically and are commonly added to moisturisers in an attempt to keep the skin soft and smooth. However, as with all nutritional supplements, lecithin is far more effective when taken internally in the form of unrefined oils. Lecithin supplements can also be taken in capsule form, derived from polyunsaturated unrefined soybean oil. However, lecithin granules and powder should be avoided as these are commonly made from egg yolk, which contains cholesterol and, due to the manufacturing process, is also likely to be oxidised (rancid), making it even more undesirable. All lecithin supplements should be taken fresh; some are protected from heat and light by a gelatine capsule coating.

How lecithin works

Lecithin also works as a lipotropic agent, that is to say it attracts fat and holds it in suspension in the blood. It functions as an edible detergent by breaking up larger fat deposits, such as cholesterol, into smaller droplets and emulsifying them so that they can be removed from the body. This prevents fatty deposits from infiltrating the liver and other vital organs and clogging up the system. It can also help prevent the arteries from becoming hardened and blocked and is therefore an important factor in the fight against heart disease and strokes.

The emulsifying action of lecithin also prevents gall stones and kidney stones by dissolving them as they form, and research suggests that lecithin also increases our resistance to disease by assisting the thymus gland which controls the body's immune system. In addition, lecithin is essential for health because it provides choline (needed for nerve impulse transmission to the brain) and inositol (needed to prevent an accumulation of fats in the liver and to maintain healthy hair). Lecithin itself is a component of the myelin sheath that surrounds nerves and may benefit sufferers of multiple sclerosis by preventing further degeneration of nerve fibres. It has been reported that many other conditions have improved with lecithin supplementation, including high blood pressure, Alzheimer's disease and senile dementia.

Lecithin for clearer skin

Lecithin is especially useful for the skin because it helps to remove the build-up of saturated fatty acids that leads to spots and other skin disorders, including acne. Many skin disorders, such as acne, blackheads, whiteheads and some dry skin conditions, are due to fatty acid degeneration in the skin's dermis. These fatty acids are mostly of animal origin, such as fatty meat, cheese and cream, as well as from hydrogenated vegetable oils which behave in the body in a similar way to saturated fats. The blocking of the dermis by these fats encourages stagnation and infection, and does not allow the free flow of the essential nutrients that the skin needs in order to thrive. Acting as an internal cleanser, the lecithin found in plant oils helps to free these stagnant deposits and clear the skin from below. This results in a smoother, fresher complexion without any blemishes. Those who suffer from severe acne or problems with recurrent spots are strongly advised to give up saturated and hydrogenated fats, to increase the amount of plant oils in their diet, and to consider taking additional supplements of vitamins A and E and zinc. (More about the diet and its link with acne on page 51).

Sources of lecithin

As lecithin is found in all living cells it is a common constituent of food and can be found in all animal and vegetable produce. However, vegetable sources are by far the most preferable as they contain polyunsaturated fatty acids. Wheatgerm is our richest natural source and contains around 4 per cent pure lecithin, followed by soya beans which contain around 2 per cent pure lecithin. Other useful supplies can be found in peanuts, corn, oats and rice. Unrefined vegetable oils are also good sources of lecithin, although the more commonly refined cooking oils have had their supplies removed during processing and contain virtually none at all.

Exercise for Face and Body

One other skin-saver that deserves at least a brief mention here is exercise. Believe me, a 20-minute jog or a reasonably strenuous work-out will do more for your skin than any face-pack ever invented. This is because exercise brings fresh blood supplies to the skin's surface and renews its nutrient supply. It also boosts the flow of lymph that carries toxins and cellular debris away from the dermis. According to the *British Journal of Dermatology*, athletes and people who work-out daily have thicker, stronger and more flexible skin. Regular exercise, which is defined as at least three 20-minute sessions a week, brings with it many health and beauty benefits. Systematic work-outs that get progressively harder are the best way to build muscle tone, burn calories, increase body strength and improve overall fitness levels. Regular exercise also improves blood circulation and therefore increases the amount of oxygen and other nutrients delivered to cells throughout the body.

Although any kind of exercise is better than none at all, the most important form of exercise for the skin (as well as for the cardiovascular system) is aerobic, which basically means exercise that leaves you out of breath. Translated literally, aerobic means 'with air' and can be applied to any form of physical activity that makes you pant. Most of us probably associate the words 'aerobic exercise' with a dance class, but most sports – even energetic walking – can be classified as aerobic activity. Expending energy in this way forces the body to take in far more air than usual, which is then transported to the muscles that are being moved and is used to release the energy stored in foods such as carbohydrates and fats. Aerobic exercise is especially important for mobilising and breaking down saturated fatty acid deposits as these are only broken down in the presence of oxygen. In fact, studies show that aerobic activity reduces cholesterol levels, especially the damaging low density lipoprotein (LDL) blood fats that are widely recognised as the most dangerous type.

Aerobic exercise is an important adjunct to any skincare regime when carried out properly and has many lasting benefits, including stronger skin and a clearer complexion. It also encourages relaxation by reducing the signs of stress and is a tremendously powerful tonic. Aerobic exercise is a recognised treatment for fighting nervous tension, anxiety and clinical depression as it increases the production of the hormone noradrenaline and boosts the neurotransmitters that send mood-improving messages to the brain. So although we may not feel much like it at the time, a brisk walk has far more chance of dispelling a dark cloud of gloom than drowning our sorrows in a bottle of wine or a handful of tranquillisers.

How to plan your work-out

Every body has different muscle strengths and stamina levels so there is no such thing as the perfect aerobic plan for all; everyone has his or her own individual abilities and the only way to long-term fitness is with a safe, gentle and well-planned approach.

Regrettably, it is impossible to transform from couch-potato to marathon runner overnight and pretty foolish to try as any attempt would almost certainly lead to injury. Having said that, the rules for beginning aerobic activity are reassuringly easy: choose any form of physical activity that makes you slightly breathless and continue working hard at it for at least 10 minutes. As you progress you will find that it gradually takes longer each time to feel out of breath. This is the signal that you should then step up the intensity of the exercise and increase the length of time that you feel out of breath. The aim is to reach a level where you feel relatively comfortable with three aerobic sessions a week lasting for at least 20 minutes each.

Contrary to popular belief, there are no age limits or restrictions to aerobic exercising, provided it is carried out safely and sensibly. Professional instructors are right to insist on a gentle warm-up and wind-down period before and after every session as this reduces the risk of potential muscle damage. Cushioned aerobic or sports shoes act as an essential pair of shock absorbers and reduce the stress of repeated impact on ankles and knees. Women should always wear a specially designed sports bra to stop breasts becoming saggy due to the over-stretching of the skin and supporting ligaments. The final golden rule is always *stop if you feel any pain*, anywhere in the body, and to consult a doctor, physiotherapist or osteopath if it does not go away.

Aerobic exercise ratings

The best kinds of exercise will raise your heartbeat to 80 per cent of its maximum level (200 beats per minute less your age). It should then keep it there for at least 10 minutes.

Excellent	Aerobics classes (with qualified supervision)
	Jogging (with cushioned shoes)
	Skiing (especially cross-country)
	Re-bounding or trampolining (ideal for beginners and those with joint problems)
Good	Cycling (especially up-hill)
	Rowing (unless you have a back problem)
	Swimming (perfect for everyone, including the young, old and pregnant)
	Walking (provided it is brisk and sustained, not just a brief stroll)
	Dancing (disco is better than ballroom)
Moderate	Tennis, badminton and table-tennis (playing singles is much harder work and more beneficial than doubles)
	Squash (short bursts of competitiveness are more harmful than sustained activity)
Poor	Riding (the horse benefits more than the rider)
	Golf (not at all aerobic unless you jog in-between swings)

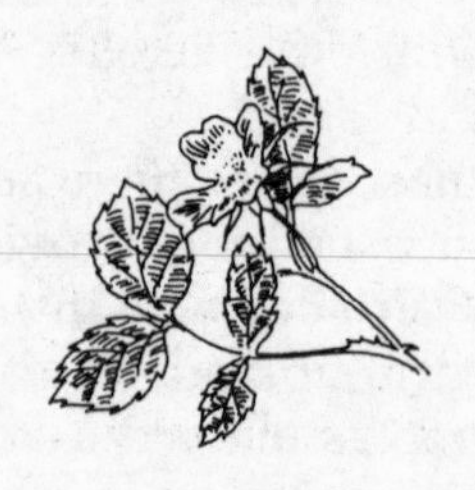

2

How To Save Your Skin

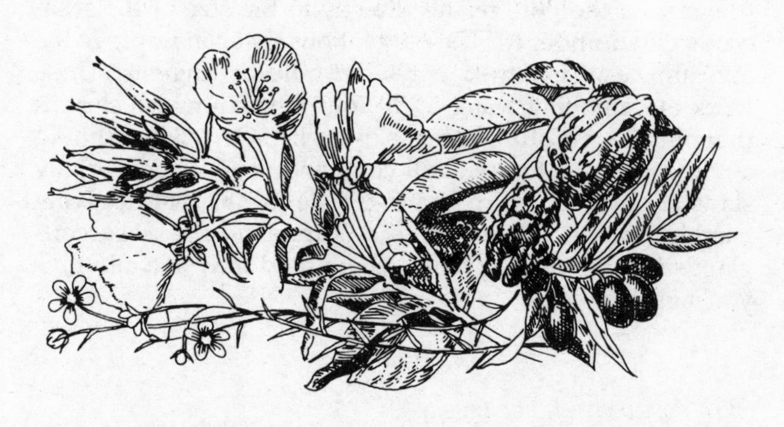

Strong, healthy, supple skin does not come out of a skincare jar but is created by the body. Despite the staggering sums spent at British cosmetic counters every year (well over £500 million on skincare, and most of this on moisturisers alone), most of us feel less than satisfied with the way our faces look and feel.

Can Skincare Products Help?

There is no doubt that we all need some form of skincare, but we do not need the over-hyped, hugely expensive and complicated regimes that are too often sold to us. Effective skincare is simple and straightforward and consists of just two fundamental factors: a cleanser to remove pollution, make-up and general grime, and a moisturising cream to protect the skin. Anything else that you choose to use might make you feel psychologically pampered but will not alter the elementary structure of your skin.

Skin toners and tonics

It is a dermatological fact of life that we do not need skin toners or tonics to remove all traces of a cleanser – warm water does the trick just as well. Despite the claims made for skin tonics, these bottles of coloured water and alcohol will *not* close your pores (the pores have no muscles so cannot contract). Large pores mean that you also have large oil glands and there is nothing that can be done to alter this (the size of the pore relates directly to the size of the sebaceous gland under it). The only lotions that can improve the appearance of enlarged pores are mild astringents. These work by removing water to dry out the skin which shrinks the plump, moisture-laden skin cells. Dry skins should avoid astringent tonics at all costs and combination or oily skins should use them sparingly. Be aware that applying harshly medicated toners can stimulate the sebaceous glands into producing more sebum, and may actually give you a greasier skin.

Skin scrubs and face masks

Exfoliating skin scrubs are sold on the basis that sloughing away the top layers of skin stimulates cell renewal and leaves the complexion looking brighter. However, there is no conclusive evidence that removing dead skin cells from the top of the skin speeds up their rate of replacement. Occasional exfoliating (not more than once or twice a week) can certainly lift a dull, sallow complexion, but it needs to be carried out extremely gently. A light buffing with a damp, soft flannel is all that is needed to dislodge any dead skin cells that insist on clinging to the surface of the skin. Over-zealous use of a scratchy skin scrub is certainly far too brutal a ritual for our fragile faces, especially for those with very fair or fine complexions. Gentleness is the key to effective skincare and cosmetic scientists now agree that any form of irritation on the skin is not only undesirable but also potentially ageing. This is because even the mildest inflammation generates free radical activity (see page 15) beneath the surface of the skin and this is recognised as the major cause of premature ageing.

Face packs and masks are also a popular part of modern skincare and can give the skin a temporary boost by tightening the skin with ingredients such as witch-hazel. These treatments can also help draw out impurities with finely ground clays such as fuller's earth. However, the effects of all face masks are at best transient and do not lead to a long-term improvement in the skin's structure.

What Will Help?

There is no question that skincare products are useful and important for maintaining healthy skin, but most are designed to treat the symptoms of our problems and ignore their underlying cause. Take car maintenance as an illustration: if the oil warning light comes on in the car we do not solve the problem by turning off the light but by re-filling the engine with oil. Similarly, when our skin indicates that it is not functioning properly we must supply it with all the ingredients it needs to run smoothly. Following the *Save Your Skin* regime will help prevent problems such as dryness and break-outs occurring in the first place, as well as effectively delaying the signs of ageing.

Saving Your Skin from Within

Beauty from within is an important message that has been largely ignored by the beauty industry whose sole aim is to sell us increasing quantities of skincare products. Despite what the advertisements lead us to believe, no skin cream is going to revolutionise your life or have more than a superficial effect on the physiological structure of your skin. No matter how much time and money you spend on your skin, it only really responds to fundamental changes in lifestyle. What you put inside your body has a far more potent effect on the complexion than anything you choose to plaster on the outside. The only way to improve your skin's appearance dramatically is to adopt a diet that feeds the cells internally, together with an effective skincare regime to cleanse and protect the skin's surface. Vital oils play an important part in saving our skin and can be adapted to benefit every skin-type. To discover how best to treat your own individual complexion, it is important first of all to understand how the skin functions and what it needs in order to thrive. Although our faces look quite different and can be a range of colours and skin-types, beneath the surface all skin looks very much the same.

Skin Structure and Type

The outer layer of skin that we see is only the tip of the proverbial iceberg and is the beginning of a complex organ that covers us from head to toe. The average adult has around 21 square feet (2 square metres) of skin, weighing about 7 lb (3.18 kg). This is twice the size of the brain, despite the fact that it never measures more than three-sixteenths of an inch (4.7 mm) thick. Generally, the thickest areas of skin are found on our palms and the soles of our feet, where the skin measures on average one-twentieth of an inch (1.2 mm) thick, though it is sometimes much thicker. Body skin measures about one-fortieth of an inch (0.6 mm) deep while the skin on the face is little more than one-two-hundredth of an inch (0.12 mm) thick. Skin is restless and continually sheds dead cells, completely rebuilding itself once every four weeks.

The daily tasks our skin copes with are daunting and, apart from the obvious job of keeping our insides together, include repelling foreign invaders, such as chemical and bacterial agents; regulating our body temperature through perspiration; secreting waste matter via the pores; manufacturing vitamin D from sunlight; and housing our senses of touch and pain. Each square half-inch (3.2 square cm) of skin is likely to contain at least 10 hairs, 100 sweat glands, 40 inches (1 metre) of tiny blood vessels and 15 sebaceous glands.

In addition to its many different functions, there are several different types of skin that cover the face and body. Our complexion has the finest skin, but the thinnest skin of all can be found on the lips, which is why they are so vulnerable to splitting and chapping in cold weather. The outer surface, or cornea, of the eyes is covered with a modified type of skin that forms a perfectly transparent windshield. The skin that covers our joints, such as elbows and knees, is loose and flexible to allow the bones and muscles beneath it to move freely, whereas the skin on our face and neck is designed to be tighter and should snap back into place when given a gentle tug.

The elastic properties of the skin are due to its supporting network of protein fibres called collagen and elastin. It is the elastin fibres in particular that allow the skin to expand and contract (for example, during pregnancy) and we must look after these if our face is not to slacken and sag. Some areas of the face are more susceptible to skin ageing than others. Our first wrinkles appear in the corners of our eyes and quickly develop into 'crows' feet' due to perpetual blinking and our habit of squinting to avoid bright lights or cigarette smoke. The skin surrounding our eyes is also especially fine and fragile as there are few sebaceous glands in this area. Although the sebaceous glands can cause greasy skin, the natural oil (sebum) that they pump on to the surface of the face is needed to keep the skin supple and waterproof.

Reflecting inner health

The skin is a remarkable organ in that it frequently changes colour and texture in response to conditions within the body. It can turn pallid, yellow, waxen, purple, ruddy, ashen, blotchy, spotty, grey or blue and become flushed, sweaty, sore or itchy in seconds. In fact, a quick glance at the face reveals a great deal about a person and can say more in an instant about our level of inner health than any medical examination. Grey shadows under the eyes invariably mean tiredness and tension, while puffiness beneath the eyes is a sign of liver and kidney problems. Spots and pimples indicate a poor diet or a sluggish lymphatic system and skin rashes are usually caused by allergies, internal imbalances and stress. Broken capillaries and tiny red veins visible on the cheeks are often the result of a diet high in caffeine, alcohol, sugar and spices, or frequent exposure to extremes of temperature.

Beauty spots and darkened, raised moles often appear at the junction of connective tissues and those who practice macrobiotics believe that the places they occur on the face correspond to meridians or parts of the body. For example, spots directly under the eyes or between the eyebrows indicate liver disorders, while those beside the nostrils are a sign of kidney and bladder disfunctions. Beauty marks situated beneath the bottom lip relate to stomach disorders, and lung problems show up as blemishes on the cheeks. What we all aspire to is a glowing complexion that reflects the good health of the rest of the body. This is why it is important to treat the body as a whole and not just the surface of the skin alone.

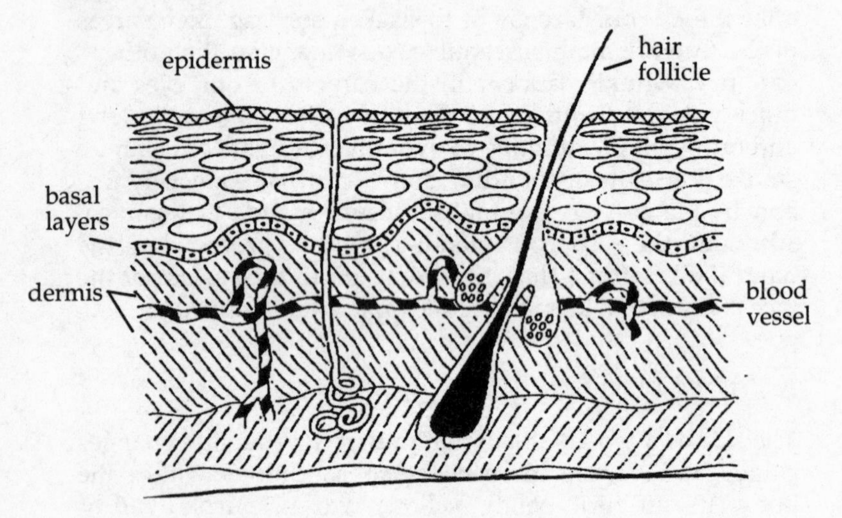

How our Skin Works

A cross-section of our skin looks a bit like a jam sandwich as it has an upper and lower layer stuck together with a fine intermediary level in between. The thin upper layer of skin is called the *epidermis*, and consists entirely of skin cells glued together with a bio-cement. The deeper, lower layer of skin comprises a fibrous network of blood vessels, nerve endings and glands, and is called the *dermis*. These two layers are separated from each other by a fine layer of skin cells known as the *basal layer*.

The epidermis is composed of four or five sheets of skin cells stuck together and it is through this that skin cells travel upwards until they reach the surface. As they rise they lose their moisture content and become thinner and stiffer. They also acquire a filling of keratin (from the Greek meaning 'horn') which makes them flat and hard. By the time they reach the skin's surface, the cells in the top layer of the epidermis are completely rigid. These hardened cells mesh together to create the outermost horny layer, or *stratum corneaum*, that protects the inner skin cells. The epidermal cells on the skin's surface are completely lifeless and the only way a moisturiser can improve their appearance is by temporarily 'glueing' the dead cells back on to the skin. A moisturiser cannot invoke a physiological change within the skin, although it can provide a film of superficial moisture that helps prevent water evaporation. Any internal moisturisation can only be achieved by adding vital oils to the diet.

As the surface skin cells die off, so they loosen and are shed in great quantities. These are then replaced by the skin cells continuously following up behind them. We shed about 4 per cent of our total number of skin cells every day and will lose around 30 lb (13.5 kg) of skin during our lifetime. The tens of thousands of skin cells that we lose every day can be found littering our homes and offices in the form of a greyish dust. In fact, all household dust is little more than dead skin cells. This continual shedding and replacement process is called cellular renewal and every anti-ageing cream ever formulated aims to speed this up to create softer, smoother skin. However, the only way to influence the rate of cellular turnover is to boost the nutrients supplied to skin cells while they are forming so that they behave in a healthier, more energetic fashion.

The activities that determine the behaviour and appearance of our skin occur deep in the depths of the dermis. This is a thick, soft cushion of connective tissue that lies beneath the epidermis. The dermis is the headquarters of all skin activity and controls what goes on above it in the epidermis and, ultimately, governs the visible appearance of the skin. In addition to its network of blood vessels, sebaceous glands, sweat glands and hair follicles, the dermis houses the connective tissue that contains the collagen and elastin fibres that support the skin.

The collagen connection

Collagen is the most abundant constituent of connective tissue and makes up around 70 per cent of the dermis. It is divided into soluble and insoluble parts; younger skin contains far more soluble collagen (also known as embryonal collagen). As we grow older, this ratio changes and we end up with more insoluble collagen which is more easily broken down, resulting in looser, sagging skin. A high proportion of older or insoluble collagen in the dermis also results in dryer, more wrinkled-looking skin.

Collagen (extracted from cow skin) is added to some moisturisers in an attempt to reinforce the skin's own supplies, but it is an enormous molecule and cannot penetrate the surface of the skin (its molecular weight is over 1 million). Some skin creams contain soluble collagen, which is a smaller molecule (around 300,000 in molecular weight) but this is still too large to slip through the epidermis. However, soluble collagen has the ability to attract and bind water, especially at low relative humidities, and is useful in creating a smooth, satiny feel on the face. The only way collagen can be put into the complexion is by injecting it directly into the dermis. Bovine collagen injections (from cow fat) are an increasingly common form of out-patient plastic surgery and aim to plump out fine lines and wrinkles. There are several side-effects to this process, however, including the risk of the collagen hardening into small visible bumps beneath the surface of the skin, not to mention the added drawbacks of the expense and the pain. Collagen injections are at best temporary and need to be repeated every few months to maintain the results. As the long-term consequences of injecting bovine collagen into the human body have not been clearly established, it is not a procedure I can recommend. A safer (and cheaper) option is to enrich the body with the ingredients that are involved with collagen production, such as the antioxidant nutrients, vitamins C and E, as well as the essential fatty acids.

Elastin

The second most important group of proteins in the connective tissue are the elastin fibres, although these only make up 5 per cent of the dermis. The elastin fibres are woven between the strands of collagen and give them additional strength and elasticity. As with collagen, elastin can be extracted from bovine fat cells but it also has a high molecular weight of over 1 million. It is usually modified, therefore, into smaller particles before being added to skin creams. However, it is still not possible for the elastin molecules to penetrate the epidermis and its value in a moisturiser is questionable.

As we age, both our collagen and elastin fibres lose their natural elasticity which basically means that our skin starts to sag and those attractive crinkles in our face and neck turn into deeper, less desirable wrinkles. The way to avoid this is to supply the dermis with all the ingredients it needs to create collagen and elastin to preserve its natural strength and elasticity.

Nourishing the skin

The skin is nourished via the rich reservoir of blood vessels that literally feed the face, and the dermis relies on an extensive network of blood vessels for a steady supply of essential nutrients. Unfortunately, the body's blood circulation does not always deliver the goods, and the skin is very sensitive to nutritional deficiencies. This is because other organs in the body take priority, and essential nutrients may be directed to other areas, such as the heart, brain and muscles, leaving the skin short-changed. The *only* way to keep the dermis healthy and strong is with optimum nutrition and this includes a daily dose of the all-important essential fatty acids, vitamin E and lecithin. Natural plant oils are the very best source of these skin-savers. These vital oils include unrefined sunflower, corn and sesame seed oils for cooking, and supplements, such as evening primrose oil and passionflower oil.

Knowing Your Skin's Needs

All skin is created more or less equal beneath the surface; it is our genetic factors and lifestyles that effect its outward appearance. Our skin colour is determined by the presence of a natural brown pigment called melanin produced by melanocytes in the epidermis. It is this pigment that gives us a suntan and determines the natural shade of the skin. The only other difference within the skin is our rate of cellular renewal, and black skins seem to shed dead skin cells faster than paler complexions, which is one reason why they tend to age more slowly.

Not only skin colour is pre-determined genetically, but tanning ability and pore size can also be attributed to heredity. There is virtually nothing we can do to change these factors; heredity is the one rogue factor in the skincare game that we have no control over. We can choose our friends but not our family. However, we can make good use of genetics by looking at the faces of our parents and grandparents to see how well they have aged. If their complexions are prematurely lined and grey, this is a warning that we will have to take extra care of our own face against the effects of time.

Hormones are also a major factor in the way our skin behaves and are responsible for pre-menstrual break-outs, adolescent acne, stretch marks during pregnancy and patches of uneven pigmentation during the menopause. While hormonal problems are tricky to treat it is possible to regulate fluctuating hormone levels and improve the skin at the same time. The essential fatty acid GLA (see page 11), found in borage and evening primrose oils, effects the production of the biological regulators (prostaglandins) that regulate many bodily functions. Although biochemists have yet to pin-point exactly how they work, prostaglandin activity is involved in many hormonal processes and has a powerful influence on the state of the skin. Large amounts of GLA, for example, have been found to help many cases of eczema and psoriasis, while doses as low as one capsule a day can reduce itchiness, skin scaling and dehydrated skin conditions. Evening primrose oil has also been found to help acne patients, probably by regulating the hormonal imbalances that lead to this chronic skin condition.

Although the internal workings of the skin are much the same, there are many different external factors that affect the way it behaves, so before deciding how to treat your complexion it is worth taking a look at your environment and living conditions. The amount of moisture in the air affects the relative dryness of the skin and, while we may not always be thankful for our inclement weather, a damp climate leads to softer, smoother skin. This is the main reason why the Irish, in particular, have such legendary complexions. Expatriates living in tropical regions are often horrified at how quickly their skins turn to shoe leather in a hot climate, simply because of a lack of moisture in the atmosphere. When you consider that moisture is the only difference between a grape and a raisin, it is easy to see why we should drink sufficient amounts of water to replenish natural moisture from within the skin. During the winter months, when our skins have their moisture content leached by central heating, it is also worth investing in a small humidifier for the home, or keeping bowls of water around the house or office.

Skin sensitivity

All skin can be sensitive, regardless of skin-type, which is why the *Save Your Skin* regime avoids common allergens and substances likely to irritate a sensitive face. However, genuinely sensitive skin is rarer than we are led to believe and most of those who fear that their skin is sensitive are worrying unnecessarily. One survey revealed that a staggering 75 per cent of all women buying skincare products believe they have sensitive skin. This high figure is not backed by dermatologists, however, who take the view that most of us fuss far too much over our faces in the first place.

Whether we're truly sensitive-skinned or not, it is still sensible to avoid known irritants. The main culprits likely to cause a reaction on the surface of the skin are alcohol, bovine collagen, colourants, camphor, detergents, lanolin, magnesium aluminium silicate, menthol, p-amino benzoic acid or PABA (a B-complex vitamin used in many sunscreen formulations), perfume and soap or soap-based cleansers. Most hypo-allergenic brands do not contain these ingredients and are made with as few ingredients as possible to minimise the overall risk of skin irritation. If your skin tends to react to new products, it is worth carrying out a patch-test on your inner arm before making a purchase. Apply a small amount of the product and leave for 24 hours. If your skin is sensitised by any of these irritants, seek out the few ranges that currently give a list of ingredients on the package, though it can be difficult, at the moment, to detect the presence of many individual ingredients as product labelling is not compulsory in Britain. However, the EC is currently reviewing this issue and we will probably find that cosmetic ingredient listing will become compulsory in Europe by the mid 1990s. Meanwhile, you could switch to an American brand which already lists its ingredients in order to comply with the Federal Drug Administration regulations in the USA. Alternatively, most skincare companies will release details of their product ingredients upon request.

Three skin slayers

In addition to the external factors that we should steer clear of, there are also a few internal elements that we must avoid in order to improve the condition of our skin. Since skin starts its life inside the body it is heavily influenced by lifestyle factors such as diet and smoking. Although we can increase our intake of essential fatty acids and other nutrients found in unrefined plant oils, their action can be blocked by three main substances: alcohol, saturated fat and smoking. In addition to preventing the skin-saving action of the vital oils, these complexion killers are also the cause of many other problems for the skin.

Alcohol:
How many heavy drinkers do you know with an enviable complexion? The answer will no doubt be none because alcohol is a fundamental enemy of the skin. No matter what your favourite tipple is, all types of alcohol encourage internal dehydration, leach much-needed moisture from the dermis and destroy the B-complex vitamins. Skin tissue consists of 20 per cent water and, as alcohol leads to dehydration, it should be avoided by those whose skin is the slightest bit dry or sensitive. Those with normal, combination or oily skin-types should at least make sure they match every alcoholic drink with an equal amount of water.

Alcohol also dilates the fragile blood vessels in the face, encouraging the tiny capillaries to expand and burst. Much of the network of broken red veins on the cheeks can be attributed to alcohol and, unfortunately, these are more visible in the fairer-skinned. Skin rashes are often triggered by the additives or chemical colourants routinely added to wine and liqueur drinks, and virtually all wine contains sulphur dioxide which is also known to cause skin blotchiness. If you want to drink alcohol on occasions, you can minimise the damage done to your skin by drinking plenty of water or diluted fruit juice and taking 500 mg of evening primrose oil plus 500 mg of vitamin C before going to bed.

Saturated fat:

It is well known that saturated fats are bad for our health but they are also hazardous for the skin. Not only do saturated animal fats interfere with our conversion of essential fatty acids but they also clog the dermis with fatty deposits that encourage bacteria-based spots. As we have seen, however, not all fat is bad for us and every skin-type benefits from replacing saturated animal fats with monounsaturated and polyunsaturated vegetable oils.

Dairy produce is notoriously high in saturated fats, especially cream, full-fat milk and cheese. Some people are also intolerant of the milk sugar called lactose due to an enzyme deficiency, and they may experience dairy-related skin disorders. Others may find that they cannot tolerate milk proteins and that these trigger skin rashes or asthmatic symptoms. Avoiding this group of dairy products has paid dividends to sufferers of many skin conditions as diverse as acne and eczema. However, it is important to keep your calcium intake high by switching to calcium-enriched soya milk, and to eat plenty of sesame and sunflower seeds, nuts (notably almonds), broccoli and root vegetables. Those who find that their skin improves if they omit most cows' milk products from their diet may be able to tolerate low-fat yoghurt and goats' milk.

Smoking:

No one these days needs to be told about the dangers of smoking and we must all be aware by now that cigarettes are a major killer. However, those looking for further incentive to kick the poisonous weed may also like to know that smoking slaughters your skin as quickly as it destroys the lungs. As well as causing chronic dehydration, smoking also force-feeds the skin with ready-made free radicals (see page 15). American studies into the premature ageing of women smokers have found that there are few more effective ways of creating wrinkles than smoking. The benzopyrene in tobacco smoke blocks the body's absorption of vitamin C and damages the collagen fibres that support the skin. Smoking also wipes out the skin-saving nutrient vitamin E, needed to repair skin tissues and prevent the visible signs of skin ageing. Smokers have a typically grey, pallid complexion due to cigarette smoke causing the blood vessels in the dermis to contract, restricting the levels of available nutrients delivered by the bloodstream. Unfortunately, even those who do not smoke may still suffer from the effects of 'passive' smoking; scientists have established that the free radicals and other carcinogens found in the sidestream of smoke from a cigarette is more dangerous than the substances inhaled by the smoker. If smoke gets up your nose it is well worth taking additional supplements of the anti-oxidant vitamin C and vitamin E to help mitigate the free-radical damage triggered within the skin. Better still, make your home a smokeless zone or negotiate a smoke-free area in the office.

Knowing Your Skin-type

Lifestyle and environment largely determine the state of your skin and which skin-type you have. Although most of us are likely to know whether our skin is dry, combination or oily, it is worth noting that because our skin is constantly changing, so our skin-type also alters. Those with dry skins will find that their complexions improve in the summer months as humidity levels increase and there is more moisture in the atmosphere. On the other hand, dryer skin conditions are aggravated during the winter when we live indoors with the central heating on full blast. Similarly, sebum levels also fluctuate according to factors such as diet and hormonal changes, so the state of an oily or combination complexion is likely to change fairly frequently. Determining the current condition of your skin is straightforward as it depends almost entirely on sebum production. You can usually judge your skin-type simply by scrutinising your face under a strong, unflattering light, but those who remain unsure can try these slightly more scientific methods of analysis.

The tissue test

Before washing your face in the morning, take a paper tissue and gently press it against your face. Hold it in place for half a minute or so, then hold it up to the light. If it is completely clean, your skin is dry and possibly sensitive. If it has a very light imprint of sebum, you have normal skin. If it has left a clear T-zone imprint of sebum from the nose and forehead, then you have a combination skin-type. If you discover a complete, clear face-print it will come as no surprise to learn that you have an excessively oily complexion.

The tape test

Remove any make-up and stick a piece of clear Sellotape across your nose. Press firmly before whisking it off and examining it under a bright light. Those with dry, mature skins will find tiny flakes of skin attached to the tape and will notice a dense, even speckling of dead skin cells. Those with combination or oily skins will see the imprints of enlarged pores in visibly uneven patches. The oilier the skin, the blotchier the marks on the tape will be, due to increased sebum production.

Magnifying measures

A magnifying mirror is essential for expertly applied make-up and will also reveal the final clues in determining skin-type. Examine your freshly cleaned face in a bright light to see which category your complexion falls into.

Dry/mature: Very fine pores; texture is dull and lifeless; shows signs of fine lines and premature wrinkles; tend to itch and flake; prone to rashes (see page 42)

Normal: Even sized, small pores; no spots, white-heads or blackheads; no sign of dryness or flakiness; rosy cheeks and a general glow (see page 54)

Combination: Visible pores on nose and chin; shiny panel on nose and forehead; blackheads on nose; possible whiteheads around cheeks and eyes (see page 47)

Oily/acne: Obviously enlarged pores; thick texture, often sallow coloured; shiny in most places; acne or severe spots, whiteheads and blackheads; few facial lines or wrinkles (see page 50)

Having established which skin-type you are, turn to the relevant section of this chapter and follow the guidelines on saving your own skin. Although the routines are similar, each have significant differences, so it is important to assess your current skin-type correctly from the start. After just one month of following the *Save Your Skin* regime you will see a significant improvement in your complexion. After three months you will have encouraged your skin to behave in a more 'normal' fashion and can then go on to the guidelines for normal skin-types on page 54. These are designed to maintain your youthful, glowing complexion and keep your face in great shape for the rest of your life.

Dry and Mature Skin-types

Those with dry and more mature complexions will find comfort in the knowledge that this skin condition responds more quickly than any other to the vital oils treatment. There are many factors that affect dry skin and diet is one of the easiest to change. All skin cells are surrounded by a protective oil (lipid) membrane which contains essential fatty acids such as GLA (see page 11). The lipidic barrier in the epidermis that prevents moisture loss also contains linoleic acid. It is clear that these essential fatty acids are extremely important for preventing dryness and overall dehydration.

Other nutrients useful in treating dry skin conditions include several vitamins. A scaly skin may be an indication of vitamin A deficiency, especially if the skin is rough and dry on the hips, knees, elbows and backs of the upper arms. Slackening skin can also be a sign that you are short of vitamin C which is needed to maintain strong, resilient collagen. Dermatological studies reported in *The Lancet* and *The British Journal of Dermatology* have also found that those with dry skins have shown deficiencies of the EPA and DHA (see page 13) essential fatty acids found in fish oils.

Dry skin is the most vulnerable to wrinkling and has the disadvantage of looking prematurely aged, making you appear old before your time. Older skin itself has the problem of increased sensitivity and is far more fragile than young skin because it lacks the more youthful soluble collagen that keeps the skin strong. More mature skins are also prone to broken capillaries and tiny red veins appearing on the cheeks and nose. In addition to regular or excessive alcohol intake, these are also caused by sudden changes in temperature, so avoid saunas, facial steams and washing your face with very hot or ice-cold water. Mature complexions also suffer from severe moisture loss as the lipidic barrier breaks down with age, and precious water escapes from the skin.

Internal skincare for dry and mature skin-types

Watching what we eat is a fundamental part of improving dry skin conditions and reversing the visible signs of ageing. Saturated fats are very damaging to dry skin as they block the body's natural conversion of linoleic acid to GLA. Without this essential fatty acid our skin cells weaken, their protective membranes lose internal moisture and the skin rapidly becomes devitalised. Saturated fats also clog the blood vessels that feed the skin and lower the levels of nutrients available to the dermis for maintaining a glowing complexion. Simply by substituting vital vegetable oils for saturated animal fats in our diet will significantly improve all dry skin problems.

Increasing the amount of unrefined plant oils in your diet is straightforward and quickly becomes a way of life. You do not need to use much oil to see a visible improvement in your skin's texture – just one tablespoonful each day is all that is needed to re-moisturise the skin from within. Try using cold-pressed olive oil for frying instead of butter or lard, and use liberal amounts of home-made salad dressings made with unrefined sunflower or safflower oils. Many delicious oil-enriched recipes can be found on pages 122 to

145, or try experimenting by adding unrefined oils to your favourite recipes.

Apart from the essential fatty acids, the other nutrients needed to improve dry skin conditions include beta-carotene (ensure a daily dose of 5–15 mg), vitamin E (naturally present in unrefined oils) and lecithin (also found in unrefined oils). Lecithin also has the ability to lock moisture into the skin so it is especially useful for dry skin conditions; those with severely dehydrated complexions should supplement their diet with one or two lecithin capsules a day. Oil supplements are also beneficial for all dry skin conditions and a daily capsule of borage or avocado oil will noticeably speed up the internal re-moisturising process. Eating more oily fish, such as mackerel and herring, also supplies drier skins with the EPA and DHA essential fatty acids that they need. Alternatively, take a daily dose of cod liver oil or fish oil.

In addition to watching what they eat, those with drier skins must also keep an eye on their drinks. Alcohol is an obvious no-no as it dehydrates the skin from within and increases the risk of skin dryness. Stimulants, such as caffeine, can also aggravate broken veins, so switch to drinking decaffeinated coffee or herbal teas for the sake of your skin as well as your nervous system. Filtered water is the best choice of all, as this screens heavy metals such as lead and aluminium as well as the disinfectant chlorine routinely added to tap water. Some bottled waters may also be useful but many contain large amounts of sodium (salt) which will also dehydrate the skin from within. Always check that the brand you buy has a low sodium content before drinking it on a regular basis.

External skincare for dry and mature skin-types

The most important part of all external skincare is thorough and efficient cleansing. Although Cleopatra chose asses' milk and Mary Queen of Scots rinsed her face in red wine, the most popular form of cleansing remains washing with soap and water. However, if your skin is dry, mature or sensitive this is the last kind of cleansing that you should opt for. Soap is strongly alkaline and easily upsets the skin's naturally acidic protective film that sits on the surface of the skin. Those with oilier skin-types can get away with using a cleansing bar or facial wash that matches the skin's natural pH value, but drier skin-types need a more emollient form of cleanser. Soap has other drawbacks, too, as it cannot dissolve make-up (which is oil-based), does not deep clean the pores, and cannot remove the build-up of sebum that leads to spots and blackheads.

Everyone with a dry skin needs an oil-based cleanser and the most versatile cleanser of all is a pure plant oil. Natural oils such as johoba oil, almond oil or peach kernel oil are useful for removing all types of make-up (especially stubborn waterproof mascara) and will gently dissolve sebum, dirt and cellular grime. Simply massage a few drops into dry skin before removing with pads of cotton wool dampened with hand-hot water, or a flannel wrung out in hot water. Never use paper tissues to cleanse dry or sensitive skin as they are made from wood pulp and contain tiny particles of bark that can scratch and upset the skin. Face flannels should be washed regularly in a non-biological detergent that is less likely to leave traces of potentially troublesome silicate residues on the skin. Baby oil should not be used on the face. This by-product of the petroleum industry contains synthetic fragrance and has no natural nutrients to enrich it.

Although skin tonics and toners are not necessary to remove all traces of oil-based cleansers, those who live in hard water areas may find that their tap water leaves a fine layer of scum on both the skin as well as the rim of the basin. This can be removed from the face with a camomile floral water, made by infusing a camomile tea bag in a jug of freshly boiled bottled water. Leave for a few minutes while the herbal infusion steeps before removing the bag and bottling the fluid. As this blend contains no preservatives, it should be stored in the fridge and used within a few days. Camomile water can be used by sprinkling a few drops on to a pad of cotton wool and sweeping over the face, or decanted into a small purse-spray or indoor plant mister and lightly sprayed over the face.

Occasional exfoliation is also useful for dry skins to buff away the dead skin flakes that tend to accumulate on the drier areas of the face. Several natural foods make good exfoliants for dry and mature skins, including finely ground oatmeal mixed with yoghurt or milk, or ground almonds made into a paste with a few drops of water. These are especially beneficial as they release traces of nourishing almond oil when rubbed gently over the skin.

Keeping the skin well moisturised is the second golden rule for dry and mature skins. Although moisturisers are essential they need not be expensive and natural plant oils work as well as the more expensive skin serums. Avocado oil is extremely nourishing (it is a useful source of lecithin) and is easily absorbed. Wheatgerm oil is the richest of all plant oils and has the highest vitamin E content. Both can be found in good health food shops and a few drops smoothed over the cheeks and gently tapped around the eye area make a very effective anti-ageing treatment for repairing damaged skin and delaying the formation of fine lines and wrinkles. As wheatgerm oil is thicker and stickier than most oils, it is advisable to use it only as a night-time treatment just before going to bed. Water sprays are also useful for replenishing the skin with moisture and should be used frequently if you live or work in a centrally heated or air-conditioned environment.

A word about eczema

Unfortunately, those with dry skin conditions are also more likely to suffer from skin disorders such as eczema and psoriasis. These conditions are notoriously difficult to treat, and as yet there is no cure, but many patients can control their condition by increasing the levels of essential fatty acids in their diet. A diet enriched with the essential fatty acid GLA (see page 11) helps many sufferers rid their skin of all symptoms and can miraculously replace itchy, swollen sores with smooth, supple skin. On a personal note, I have successfully treated my own eczema for many years by taking a daily dose of GLA and only suffer a flare-up when I forget to take it. Borage oil is the richest source of GLA for those who want to try it, or you can take evening primrose oil which is available on prescription from your GP to treat atopic eczema. This is the commonest type of eczema in childhood and evening primrose oil is clinically well-documented as being beneficial. As well as adding daily doses of essential fatty acids to the diet, eczema sufferers are also likely to benefit from excluding all dairy products from their diet. When bathing, it is also important to avoid harsh soaps and detergent-based bath foams (emollients from the chemist are amongst the gentlest cleansers) and to add a few drops of almond oil to the water to soothe irritated skin. Lastly, moderate amounts of sunshine also help many eczema sufferers, so get a daily dose of fresh air – but do not forget your facial sunblock (see page 67).

Combination Skin-types

If you have a combination skin-type you are not alone as this is the most common skin condition and reflects a complexion that is struggling to cope with a conflict of internal and external elements. On the one hand, extreme oil production by the sebaceous glands, especially around the nose, forehead and chin areas, is aggravated by hormonal factors and excessive saturated fat in the diet. On the other hand, environmental factors such as central heating, air conditioning and dehydrating skincare products, such as medicated toners, combine to dry out the skin, leading to dullness and flakiness.

Those with combination skin often feel as though they are dealing with two separate faces, as the skin condition of areas such as the cheeks and chin are very different. Combination skin is typified by a shiny nose which tends to 'creep' through make-up, making it difficult for foundation to stay in place. The short-term answer for this is to carry a powder-compact with you and to 'blot' the sebum with translucent pressed powder as it starts to appear on the nose and chin. The longer term solution, however, requires a little more forethought.

It's not all bad news, however, and those with combination complexions can take heart that because their skin is producing more sebum than most it is also well-lubricated and less prone to developing premature lines and wrinkles. The drawback of producing excess sebum is that you are also more likely to have spots, pimples and blackheads. This is due to a build-up of sebum forming a hard plug over the entrance to a pore or hair follicle. This plug leads to a build-up of sebum and fatty deposits beneath the surface of the skin. Blackheads (comedones) are formed by a combination of the plug oxidising (reacting with oxygen in the air) which turns it black, and also by the increase in the skin pigment called melanin. In addition, boils are also a common problem for combination skin-types and are caused when germs infect a hair follicle that has become clogged with sebum. As well as having spots and blackheads, combination complexions are typically dull, sallow or lifeless and may have visible flakes of dead, dry skin clinging to the cheeks, temples and around the eyes. Fortunately, all these factors can easily be remedied.

Internal skincare for combination skin-types

Re-balancing the amount of sebum produced by the sebaceous glands in the skin is the most important part of coping with combination skin. As we have seen, saturated fats in the diet block the body's process of converting linoleic acid into the essential fatty acid GLA (see page 00) that regulates hormonal activity. Imbalances in prostaglandins, the biological regulators in the body, frequently lead to excessive sebum production, so a daily dose of a GLA-enriched oil, such as evening primrose oil or borage oil, can help. Hormonal changes also occur after taking the contraceptive pill, becoming pregnant or going on to hormone replacement therapy (HRT). A daily dose of GLA may help prevent the results of these unusual imbalances becoming visible in the skin. Far from making the skin oilier, a daily dose of vital oils can help regulate the skin's natural sebum production.

External skincare for combination skin-types

Unlike dirt and general dead-cell debris found on the surface of the face, blackheads and boils cannot simply be washed away. The fundamental rule with all types of spots is not to touch them with your fingers. This leads to cross-infection and the grease and grime on even the cleanest-looking finger will only feed the ever-hungry bacteria. It is also important not to squeeze any spot as the skin is designed to be a self-healing organ and attempts to disrupt the healing process can delay it further and encourage infection. Some beauty therapists also maintain that squeezing a spot or blackhead can permanently twist the pore and trap the sebum beneath it. There is no doubt that while squeezing a spot will work temporarily, it eventually interferes with the pore's own ability to expel waste-matter and can lead to more severe skin problems.

The best way to combat blackheads is gently to dissolve the hardened plug of sebum that is blocking the pore. One of the most effective methods of doing this is to dab pure alcohol (available from chemists) on to the blackheads, using a fresh cotton bud for each one. Other useful solvents include vodka (so imagine what it does for your insides) and acetone (found in cheaper nail varnish removers and also available from chemists). Boils and other infected spots respond well to a regular dab of naturally antiseptic lavender essential oil, available from most health food shops and chemists that sell aromatherapy ranges.

Keeping the skin free from excessive sebum is obviously critical to prevent spots and blackheads from recurring, and cleansing is the most important part of your skincare routine. The best way to reduce oil on the surface of the skin is with an oil-based cleanser. This is because oil dissolves best in oil, not water. You can easily make your own cleanser simply by rubbing a few drops of sweet almond oil, johoba oil or grapeseed oil on to the face and neck. Add a single drop of antiseptic lavender oil if spots are a problem. Remove the oil with pads of cotton wool dampened with hand-hot water or a clean face flannel wrung out in hot water (wash after each use). You do not need to use a skin toner, but if you live in a hard-water area and find that the water tends to leave a scum around the rim of the basin, you can use a mild home-made astringent based on diluted cider vinegar to restore the skin's natural pH balance (this will also help to disguise the appearance of enlarged pores). Dilute one teaspoonful of good quality cider vinegar in a tumbler of bottled water before using on the face.

Moisturisers are useful, not only on the driest parts of the face but also on the oilier areas, as the dehydration that leads to lines and wrinkles is caused by the amount of *water* in the skin, not the levels of oil. If you use a plant oil cleanser you will find that the oil penetrates through to the upper layers of the epidermis and you may not need to add a moisturiser at all. However, if the cheeks and eye areas of your face are very dry you can use a few drops of cold-pressed avocado or hazelnut oil directly on the skin before going to bed. Both avocado oil and hazelnut oils are quickly absorbed into the skin, but should be used sparingly.

Oily and Acne Skin-types

Those with excessively greasy skin may curse their over-enthusiastic sebum secretions but can take heart in the knowledge that oilier skins are better protected from the onslaughts of the elements. However, it is a sad fact that most of those with very oily skin also suffer from some form of acne. Over 70 per cent of teenagers are estimated to have acne at any one time, although most of this is classified as mild acne which clears within 12 months. About 10 per cent suffer from moderate acne which can last several years, while 3 per cent of those afflicted suffer severe acne until their thirties. Acne is not only a teenage condition, however, and it is not uncommon for it to strike us for the first time when we are in our twenties.

Very oily skin and acne are both caused by the same contributing factor: excessive sebum production. The amount of sebum (the skin's natural oil) produced by the sebaceous glands is controlled by a group of male hormones known as androgens. The main androgen responsible for regulating sebum output is testosterone, a hormone found in both men and women. It is an imbalance of testosterone during puberty, or occasionally during pregnancy, that triggers excessive sebum production. The problem with producing too much sebum is that it tends to build up and block the pores and hair follicles. If this happens, bacteria quickly multiply beneath the blockage and inflammation soon sets in. This leads to the formation of pus and the familiar yellow-headed pustule. The temptation is to scratch, squeeze or pick at these spots, but this leads to further infection and subsequent scarring.

As well as hormonal disorders, vitamin A deficiency has also been linked to the formation of blackheads (comedones) and whiteheads (milia). Lack of vitamin A can cause the surface skin cells to die off too quickly and clog the sebaceous glands and pores. This then prevents sebum from being released on to the skin's surface and results in spots. Low vitamin A levels are also known to lead to skin infections such as impetigo and boils.

Internal skincare for oily and acne skin-types

Although excessive sugar consumption has not been directly linked to spots and acne, there is no doubt that a nutrient-enriched, wholefood diet is extremely helpful in improving these skin conditions. It is also extremely important that those with acne avoid all saturated fats. As acne is commonly due to hormonal imbalances, some specialists also advise avoiding meat unless it is free-range or organically reared and guaranteed free from synthetic hormones. Many acne sufferers find that their skin improves if they avoid all dairy products in the initial weeks of treatment. This may be linked to the traces of pesticides and hormones occasionally found in cows' milk and milk products.

The most important nutrients in your diet are the essential fatty acids to strengthen skin cells, vitamin E for skin healing, lecithin for clearing the build-up of fatty waste matter beneath the skin, vitamin A and zinc for repairing the skin. Your diet should include a daily dose of evening primrose oil and cod liver oil (or blended fish oil). These will not make your skin more oily but help to re-balance the sebum production within the skin. It is interesting to note that Eskimos do not suffer from acne because of their low intake of saturated fats and high dietary levels of fish oils. Eskimos only develop acne when they move away from their homeland and adopt Western eating habits.

Acne sufferers are also likely to benefit from a daily multi-vitamin and mineral supplement programme that includes 10,000 iu vitamin A (or 5–15 mg beta carotene) and 50 mg zinc (chelated for maximum absorption). An additional lecithin capsule or two taken with meals is also helpful in the initial stages to clear away the build-up of fats that lead to bacteria-based spots. In addition, it is essential to cut completely (or at least severely restrict) elements in the diet that over-stimulate the body or interfere with nutrient absorption. In addition to saturated fats, these include refined sugars, refined flours, alcohol, spices, salt, chemical additives and caffeine. Increase your consumption of whole grains, live low-fat yoghurt, garlic and unrefined vegetable oils (see recipes on page 122 to 145). Drink plenty of filtered or bottled water, take more exercise (see page 24) and enjoy a daily dose of fresh air. Rest is also a tremendous skin rejuvenator as the skin repairs and renews itself while we sleep. The value of beauty sleep is not just an old-wives' tale; a regular eight hours each night is extremely important for saving the skin.

External skincare for oily and acne skin-types

Lack of cleanliness is not usually a factor with oily skin-types, as sufferers often spend a great deal of time scrubbing their faces with medicated products. Unfortunately, this can be just as damaging as not washing at all because over-stimulating the sebaceous glands with continual cleansing can trigger them into producing yet more sebum.

Conventional medication includes oral antibiotics which kill off all internal bacteria (both good and bad) to prevent the infections that lead to acne. The mini-contraceptive pill is also sometimes prescribed to women in an attempt to even out fluctuating hormones. Tretinoin gel (Retin-A) may also be used by dermatologists for acne, but although it appears to work well it can irritate and may have harsh side-effects on the skin. Over-the-counter products containing antiseptics or benzoyl peroxide are common, but have their drawbacks and should be used sparingly. Benzoyl peroxide is effective for clearing spots, but has irritating side-effects, may bleach the skin and is fiercely dehydrating. Studies by dermatologists in Australia, however, have found tea-tree essential oil to be as effective as benzoyl peroxide at treating acne, yet without any of the harsh side-effects. This essential oil should be used sparingly and applied by using a clean cotton bud to dab the oil on to each eruption. Tea-tree oil is a powerful healer and has natural anti-fungal and antibiotic properties, making it a useful all-round antiseptic. It can be found in most health food shops and chemists that stock ranges of aromatherapy essential oils.

Cleansing the skin is important, but conventional soaps

are highly alkaline and do not dissolve sebum. The answer is to choose pH-balanced cleansing bars for the bath or shower and to cleanse the face twice daily with an oil-based cleanser. It may sound strange, but the best way to remove oil from the face is with an oil. This is because sebum dissolves in oil, not water, and most natural plant oils work well on oily skins, including peachnut, apricot kernel or johoba oil. It is worth buying a high quality oil that has not been extracted with synthetic solvents and cold-pressed varieties can be found in good health food shops. Lightly massage a small amount of oil into the skin and remove with pads of cotton wool dampened with hand-hot water, or a clean flannel wrung out in hot water (be sure to wash well after each use to prevent re-infection). The warmth from the hot water stimulates the flow of blood to the face and helps speed the healing process. Pat the skin dry with a soft towel that is washed after each use. Oil cleansers are also highly efficient make-up removers and small amounts can safely be used to remove even the most stubborn waterproof mascaras. Baby oil should not be used on the face, however (see page 45). A cider vinegar astringent tonic may be used after cleansing to help disguise the appearance of enlarged pores. Dilute one tablespoonful (or more in extreme cases) of good quality cider vinegar in a tumbler of bottled water and apply with cotton wool.

Regular exfoliating to clear the debris from the surface of the skin and unclog the pores is also a useful treatment for oily skins, although gentleness is the key to avoid overstimulating the sebaceous glands. One of America's leading dermatologists and cosmetic surgeons, Dr Lewis Feder, recommends that his patients use refined white sugar mixed with a little water as a natural exfoliant. He maintains that the granules are just the right size for loosening debris trapped in the pores and that oily skin in particular benefits from the sugar's slightly anti-bacterial properties (when applied externally, not when eaten!). If you have fine, fragile skin, use caster sugar, otherwise granulated sugar is suitable. However, do not scrub any area of 'active' acne or skin blemishes. Contrary to popular belief, moisturisers are also important for oily skins, as it is the *water* content and not the *oil* content of the skin that causes dryness and premature ageing. Those who use oil cleansers will find that their skin becomes naturally softer as the oil automatically penetrates and moisturises the upper layers of the epidermis. Any other areas of dryness can be treated with a few drops of the lightest plant oils, such as johoba or apricot kernel oil.

Normal Skin-types

Congratulations! You have either been following the *Save Your Skin* plan for several weeks, or else you already lead a naturally blameless lifestyle. Of course, you could also have inherited a perfect skin as part of your genetic make-up. This regime is designed not only to keep normal skin healthy but also to delay the signs of ageing. A normal skin-type is not only something to aspire to, it is a condition we can all achieve by following the guidelines in this book. Plant oils are powerful healers and combined with a sensible skincare and diet plan, are a foolproof method of achieving a better-looking skin.

Internal skincare for maintaining normal skin-types

Caring for the skin from within is as important as preventing the signs of premature ageing with external skincare. The healing effects of nutrients, such as the essential fatty acids and vitamin E, are well documented, and we have already seen in the previous chapter just how valuable these internal skin-savers are. A balanced diet, enriched by vital oils, is a fundamental factor in preserving your face and warding off wrinkles. This is why you will find many delicious oil-enriched recipes on pages 122 to 145, together with guidelines for easy ways to include a small amount of oil in your food every day. Remember to use only unrefined cooking oils as these retain their natural levels of vitamin E and lecithin, and will help to improve the condition of your skin. Many of the beauty oil supplements also help delay the effects of time on the skin and a daily dose of passionflower oil or evening primrose oil will help to maintain overall smoothness and elasticity.

External skincare for maintaining normal skin-types

The main concern when looking after normal skin is to keep it soft, supple and strong. We also want to delay the visible signs of ageing and prevent common sub-surface skin damage from occurring in the dermis. Thorough cleansing is important to keep the skin free from surface dirt and bacteria, and to keep the production of sebum flowing smoothly. Oil-based cleansers are the most efficient form of cleansing the skin, removing make-up and stubborn grime. Pure plant oils, such as johoba or almond oil, can also be used as economical cleansers by rubbing a few drops into the skin and removing with pads of cotton wool dampened with hand-hot water or a face flannel wrung out in hot water (always wash after each use). As oil cleansers also penetrate the upper layers of the skin they tend to leave the skin sufficiently soft and moisturised. However, those living or working in dehydrating environments can reinforce their superficial moisture levels by massaging a few drops of avocado, wheatgerm or johoba oil directly on to the skin as a nourishing night-time treatment. Whatever type of treatments you choose, remember that skincare does not stop at the chin but should continue over the entire throat as well. Your neck needs just as much nourishment as your face and few things give the age game away faster than a wrinkled, crêpey-looking neck.

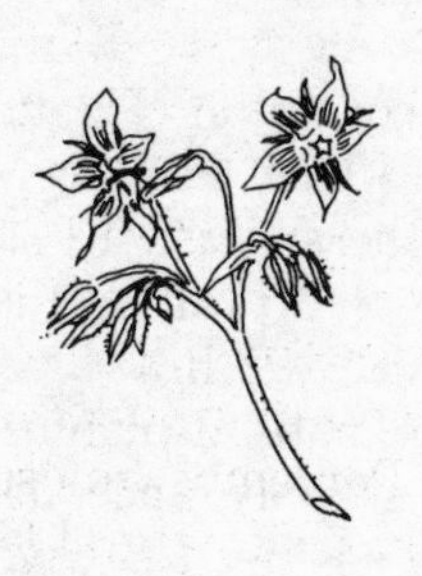

3

The Vital Oils

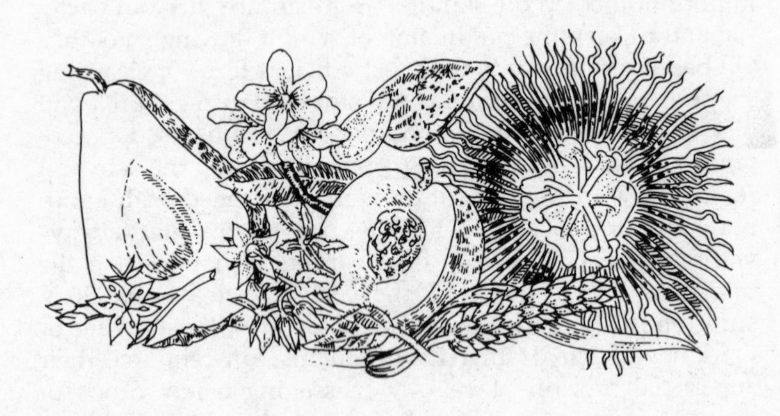

As we have seen, the essential fatty acids found in natural oils are powerful skin-savers and the beauty of them is that they are all so easy to use. The golden rule is simply to add a few drops of these vital oils to your diet every day. Their effect within the body is dramatic as they work by immediately strengthening every skin cell in the body. You will see the difference in the condition of your skin after only a few weeks of regular use. They also replenish moisture levels, and reinforce suppleness, elasticity, texture and tone, and because they have such a profound effect on the skin they are also very economical. As little as one capsule or a single tablespoonful of pure, natural plant oil is all that is needed to improve the skin's appearance. Those concerned about consuming extra calories need not worry either, as oil capsules contain only 5 calories each and a tablespoonful of oil, such as olive oil, has the same calorific value as a digestive biscuit (only it is far better for you!).

Although we only need a small amount of vital oils in our diet, the risk of over-dosing on oil supplements is a common and sensible question. Fortunately, the answer is reassuring as there is no possible toxicity from taking even ridiculously large doses of plant oils. The only slight side-effect to swallowing, say, a whole bottle of almond oil would be a dramatic case of diarrhoea!

How to Use the Vital Oils

Including natural oils in your diet every day is very straightforward. One way is to make sure your kitchen is well stocked with unrefined or cold-pressed vegetable oils. These could include olive, sunflower, safflower, sesame seed, hazelnut and walnut oils. Make sure the labels state that the oils are either cold-pressed or unrefined as this ensures that they still retain their levels of important natural nutrients.

Each type of cooking oil has its own unique flavour and can be used in many different ways to maximise its beauty benefits. Descriptions and uses for these cooking oils can be found on page 117, together with many delicious, nutritious oil-enriched recipes.

However, perhaps the easiest way to ensure you receive your daily dose of the outstanding essential fatty acids is to take a regular beauty oil supplement. Since oil research first started at the beginning of this century, our choice of supplements has increased dramatically. While they are all a convenient source of skin-strengthening nutrients each is subtly different and it is worth noting their individual properties and characteristics.

Almond oil

One of the earliest cosmetic ingredients, almond oil has been used for several thousands of years to soften and soothe the skin. Its light, emollient texture has made it an essential element of heavy-duty moisturisers, especially hand and nail preparations. One of the easiest and also most effective treatments for rough, chapped hands is simply to massage a few drops of almond oil into the hands and nails before going to bed. Slipping on a pair of cotton gloves seals in the body's natural warmth and greatly increases the penetration of the oil, so by the morning the hands are silky smooth. Almond oil is also a great nail-strengthener and a few drops massaged daily around the cuticles improves nail growth and reinforces the natural oils within the layers of nail plate to prevent splitting and breakage. Although almond oil is an important ingredient for the beauty industry today it is probably more useful when taken internally than simply rubbed on to the skin.

Almond oil comes from almonds harvested from the sweet almond tree and is also known as 'sweet almond oil'. Almonds themselves are a useful source of vitamin E, the B vitamins, calcium, potassium, zinc and iron. As with all nuts, they also contain high levels of compounds called protease inhibitors and polyphenols that are known to stop cancerous growths in laboratory animals, and nuts are even seen by some medics as one of many possible food antidotes to cancer.

Almonds are an excellent source of natural oil and cold-pressing yields up to half their weight in almond oil. However, most of the valuable nutrients are subsequently lost during the oil refining process. Recent studies show that both almonds and almond oil can significantly help in the fight against heart disease. Studies in America have shown that those eating an almond and almond oil-enriched diet for 4 weeks had an average drop in their cholesterol levels of 11 per cent. This compares with 5 per cent for those who ate an olive and olive oil-based diet.

Whole, raw almonds make tasty snacks and should be bought in their shells, or at least complete with skins, for maximum nutritional benefit. As a result of their high oil content, all nuts, including almonds, go rancid fairly rapidly when exposed to heat and light. Ideally, all nuts should be shelled just before use or, if pre-shelled, they must be stored in an airtight container or in the fridge. Delicious recipes containing raw almonds can be found on pages 134 and 136. Ground almonds also contain useful amounts of oil (you can make your own in a coffee grinder for a fresher flavour) and are tasty additions to liven up plain low-fat yoghurt or fromage frais.

Almond oil contains 20 per cent linoleic acid which makes it a good internal beauty oil and 70 per cent monounsaturated (oleic) fatty acids, so it is also useful for cooking. It is highly versatile and can be taken in capsule or liquid form. Chemists sell purified almond oil which is both bland and fragrance-free, so you may prefer to use this directly on the skin. Some supermarkets now stock almond oil as a gourmet cooking oil for its sweet, subtle flavour, although its high price means that it is best kept for superior salad dressings and sauces.

Avocado oil

Avocado oil was one of the first oils ever used because it is so easy to extract. The avocado contains around 30 per cent pure oil which is easily released by simple mechanical pressing and filtering. Avocado oil was originally used in its native Mexico and Arizona where it was prized for cooking, as a medicine, a massage oil and even an aphrodisiac. Nutritionally speaking, the avocado is an unusually complete fruit which contains both protein and carbohydrate, as well as its fabulously rich monounsaturated oil. Avocados are also a good source of many nutrients, including beta carotene, the B vitamins (notably folic acid), and vitamins C and E. They also contain many minerals, including magnesium, potassium and iron. Although high in fat, avocados and avocado oil do not contain any cholesterol and may be enjoyed by the health-conscious.

Today, avocado oil is stilly highly regarded by the cosmetics industry as it has superb powers of penetration and skin regeneration. It is a highly nourishing plant oil and so suits severely dry and dehydrated skins, and yet it is also the most easily absorbed. More importantly, avocados have a powerful effect on the skin when taken internally and recent research has shown that substances in the pulp seem to trigger deoxyribonucleic acid (DNA) into producing soluble collagen (see page 33). A daily supplement of avocado oil is also one of the best ways to prevent dryness and skin dehydration. In addition, avocado oil is also a useful supplement to take after sunbathing (see page 67) because it helps repair skin cell membranes damaged by ultra-violet light.

Avocados have been given a hard time by dieters because they are relatively high in calories (although half an avocado chopped into a salad provides fewer calories than a portion of egg mayonnaise or cheese) and it is time that this delicious tropical fruit was reprieved. Although avocados are high in fat, they contain the beneficial monounsaturated (vegetable) oils which make them positively good for us. Intriguing studies in the United States have revealed that eating avocados as part of a low-fat diet reduces your risk of heart disease even more than switching to a low-fat diet alone. Two groups of women were monitored over a three-week period: the first were simply given a diet low in saturated animal fats, the second ate the same low-fat foods but added avocados. At the end of the trial, doctors found that the serum cholesterol levels of those who had eaten the plain low-fat diet had dropped by 4.9 per cent, but the cholesterol levels of those who also ate the avocados had fallen by a staggering 8.2 per cent. In addition, the avocado-eaters also had a marked reduction in the particularly harmful type of blood fats called low-density lipo-proteins (LDL). Further studies have also shown that the fats in avocados are unusually easy for the stomach to digest and researchers have found a unique anti-bacterial and anti-fungal substance in the pulp. No doubt we shall be hearing more about this perfect fruit in the future.

Borage oil

Given the choice of only one plant oil supplement to save my skin and well-being, I would undoubtedly choose borage oil. Romans called borage the 'herb of gladness' and used an infusion from its leaves to treat depression. Borage has been grown in Britain for centuries and its bristly, greyish-green leaves and pale blue flowers are a familiar sight in many gardens. Although the flowers are not especially sweet-smelling, borage attracts honey bees who are drawn to its blue flowers, hence its Edwardian nickname 'beebread'. Borage is also known as the starflower, due to the pointed star shape of its flowers. It has been a favourite herbalists' tonic for centuries and remedies can be made from its leaves, roots and stalk. The seventeenth-century English herbalist, Nicholas Culpeper, described borage as being good for breastfeeding, and it has since been discovered that borage oil is the best source of the essential fatty acid GLA (see page 11), which is also present in breast milk. However, borage oil can only be extracted from the tiny black seeds contained in its seed pods after the plant's flowering has finished.

A blooming miracle

Borage oil's main claim to fame is its unusually high levels of GLA and, for this reason, it is commonly added to other oil supplements to boost their essential fatty acid supplies. Borage oil contains a staggering 25 per cent GLA, which means that it is twice as concentrated as evening primrose oil (see below). In theory, this means that you need to take half as many capsules of borage oil to have the same effect on the body, which could save you a considerable amount of money.

The GLA found in borage and evening primrose oils is vitally important for a smooth, supple and strong skin. GLA protects the skin by strengthening the cell membranes which enable the skin cells to retain their natural moisture. This fortifying action also means that our skin cells are better able to resist the attacks made by free radicals and destructive enzymes in the depths of the skin. GLA is occasionally added to skin cream in the form of borage oil or evening primrose oil, but its most effective anti-ageing action comes from taking the oils internally. GLA is also a powerful skin-healer and it is this essential fatty acid that helps many cases of eczema and psoriasis. It has also been clinically proven to help with numerous hormone-related disorders, including Pre-Menstrual Syndrome and breast pain. GLA is converted into hormone-like prostaglandins so it may also be useful in relieving the effects of depression, tension and stress.

Evening primrose oil

The evening primrose is not at all like a common primrose, but is a tall, spiky plant with vivid, egg-yolk-yellow flowers. It only blooms in the evening (hence its name) and thrives on poor soil and extreme weather conditions. The evening primrose can be traced back 70,000 years to Central America and Mexico where the North American Indian medicine-men were the first to make use of its extraordinary healing powers. They made poultices from its leaves to soothe aches and sprains and used the juice from its roots as a cough mixture. They also brewed up the plant's seed pods to make anti-inflammatory infusions. In fact, it is the seed pods of the evening primrose plant that contain the secret to its more recent success. These seeds are rich in oil and are another rare natural source of the essential fatty acid GLA. One reason why evening primrose oil is so expensive is because it takes about 2,000 tiny seeds to fill a single capsule of oil.

Evening primrose oil was originally analysed in 1919, when GLA and other essential fatty acids were discovered and identified for the first time. We now know that GLA is needed for many bodily functions, and that it can be created by the body from the linoleic acid commonly found in nuts, seeds and vegetables. However, we also know that this conversion process may be blocked by many factors of modern living, including internal pollution from smoking and external pollution from chemicals such as car fumes and stress. As a result, many of us now risk a deficiency of GLA.

The GLA found in evening primrose oil (and borage oil) is biologically important because it affects much of the enzyme activity that takes place in the body. Every biological process is triggered by the action of various enzymes, including the production of prostaglandins. As we have seen, these influence many processes, including blood pressure, digestion, stress and inflammation. About 40 prostaglandins have been identified to date, although research suggests that many more will become known in the future. Prostaglandins can be found in every cell of the body; they regulate the movement of material between individual cells and control cellular communication. This inevitably means that prostaglandins are fundamental to all biological processes. As they live for only a few seconds, prostaglandins are created on the spot as needed by the cells. This is why the body needs a steady supply of GLA to ensure that this process happens smoothly. As world-wide research into the powerful actions of prostaglandins continues, the future looks likely to reveal them as being a major force in creating good health.

Flower power

- The evening primrose plant originated in Mexico and Central America over 70,000 years ago.
- Today, growers choose from many different kinds of hybrid plants but all have been bred to provide a uniform content of gamma linolenic acid (GLA).

- Evening primrose oil is used to treat over 14 different conditions in the body, ranging from eczema to schizophrenia, Pre-Menstrual Syndrome, breast pain and alcoholism.
- There have been over 100 different medical trials involving evening primrose oil.
- Amongst the latest research into this powerful plant oil is a study being conducted at the Edinburgh Royal Infirmary for the treatment of pancreatic cancer.
- Because of the action of GLA on cell membranes, evening primrose oil and other oils containing this substance have special benefits for the skin.
- An orang-utan at London Zoo has been cured of flaking skin and a lack-lustre coat with a course of evening primrose oil!

The GLA factor

The therapeutic properties of GLA are well documented, and the use of evening primrose oil has been largely accepted by the medical community. Evening primrose oil itself currently holds two medical licences and is available on prescription from GPs to treat atopic eczema and breast pain. It must also be mentioned here that the link between evening primrose oil and epilepsy remains unproved. Evening primrose oil does not appear to induce epilepsy or provoke an attack, and epileptics may take the supplement under their doctor's guidance. Detailed descriptions of the clinical studies and medical science behind evening primrose and the other therapeutic oils can be found in my earlier book on this subject, *Vital Oils* (Vermilion, 1991).

In addition to being an intense healer, the GLA in evening primrose oil (and borage oil) is also a salient factor for improving the texture and tone of the skin. The nutritional significance of essential fatty acids, including GLA, was initially highlighted in trials involving rats fed on a totally fat-free diet. The rats quickly developed rashes and scaling patches of dry skin, and similar unfortunate symptoms have been reported by men and women on a fat-free diet. The most important message here is that a small amount of some oil or fat in the diet is essential and it comes back to the question of knowing which type to choose. Certainly a diet low in saturated animal fats has very many benefits, including significant weight loss and increased health and vitality, but it must be balanced with some plant-based essential fatty acids. Those who want to cut out all oil and fat from their cooking will be well advised to supplement their diet with one or two capsules of an oil supplement, such as evening primrose oil, to ensure they receive their daily intake of these essential fatty acids.

How much should I take?
The following dosages are those recommended by the Evening Primrose Office, a public information service that collates and distributes the latest medical findings into this supplement.

Eczema	6 × 500 mg per day
Hangover	6 × 500 mg before drinking
Breast pain	6 × 500 mg per day
Pre-Menstrual Syndrome	2 × 500 mg per day (for severe PMS) 2 × 250 mg per day (for mild PMS)
Skin, hair and general health	2 × 250 mg per day or 1 × 500 mg per day

Passionflower oil

The passionflower is native to South America and now grows all over the Mediterranean and the south of England. It is named after its bright purple-tinged flowers that represent the crucifixion or 'passion' of Christ. The flowers have a group of central filaments that resemble the crown of thorns, while the stigmata are in the shape of a cross with the stamens representing the nails. Passionflower oil is extracted from the seeds of the passionflower and contains a high percentage of linoleic acid, the parent to GLA, and it is specifically used to improve skin elasticity.

Linoleic acid acts on the skin by strengthening the lipidic barrier that separates the epidermal skin cells from the dermis. It is highly effective at preventing moisture loss and ensures that the skin cells are kept fully hydrated. The breakdown of the lipidic barrier in the skin is one of the most significant factors for premature skin ageing. If we can reinforce this barrier from within we will ensure that our skin remains smooth and strong for far longer. Prevention is obviously far better than cure and a daily dose of passionflower oil is a useful way of maintaining skin elasticity and preventing fine lines and wrinkles. However, do not despair if you think you have left it a little late as passionflower oil can even help soften and smooth the more mature skins and is undoubtedly one of nature's own anti-agers.

Peachnut oil

Peachnut oil reached Britain during the Roman occupation and comes from the *Prunus persica* peach tree which has bright pink flowers. The peach tree likes a limy soil with plenty of strong summer sunshine and thrives in hot Mediterranean countries. If the conditions are right, it is not uncommon for a peach tree to live for several hundred years. Peachnut oil is extracted from the fruit's kernel and has a light texture and slightly sweet smell. It is used by beauty therapists and aromatherapists for facial massage as its feather-weight texture does not clog the pores. It is also said to encourage the skin to secrete its own natural oil, sebum, making it a good choice for facial massage by those with dry or devitalised complexions.

Peachnut oil contains both monounsaturated and polyunsaturated fatty acids and can be taken internally to promote a glossy, shining head of hair and a healthy scalp. Peachnut oil is also an easy and effective external treatment for dry, itchy scalp conditions: try rubbing a few drops into the scalp with your fingertips just before shampooing to lift away dead flakes of skin and leave the skin softened. If you cannot find peachnut oil in a bottle, use the contents of a couple of capsules, or use apricot kernel oil instead.

Wheatgerm oil

Wheat is the major food source of the world and mankind has used wheatgerm oil for thousands of years (it can be traced back as far as 2000BC). Wheatgerm oil is extracted from the 'germ', otherwise known as the embryo or nucleus, of the wheat kernel. This potent part of the plant is packed with important vitamins (notably vitamin E), minerals and oil with many essential polyunsaturated fatty acids. The oil is extracted by warm-pressing wheatgerm kernels and this gives us our richest natural source of vitamin E.

Wheatgerm oil also contains an unusual active ingredient called octacosanol, which can also be found in other grains and alfalfa. Anecdotal evidence accumulated over a number of years suggests that this may be a very useful substance that can help increase stamina and endurance, reduce the pain of arthritis, mitigate the effects of stress, speed recovery from viral infections and heal some types of skin rash. The boldest claims for octacosanol are for increasing libido and sex drive, and American trials show that it steps up the production of semen in men and can improve fertility. Biochemist Robert Lupo speculates that octacosanol works by stimulating the pituitary gland at the base of the brain, which is known as the 'master gland' and is involved with most bodily functions, including the rate at which we age. Roasted wheatgerm contains less octacosanol and other nutrients than fresh wheatgerm, which is unfortunately more difficult to obtain. The best source is probably cold-pressed wheatgerm oil in liquid or capsule form.

Wheatgerm oil itself is thick, rich and deeply nourishing. It can be taken internally as a nutritional supplement (natural vitamin E capsules are made from wheatgerm oil) or applied directly to the skin to combat cases of severe dehydration. The drawbacks to using wheatgerm oil directly on the skin are that it does have a sticky texture and faintly earthy smell which you either love or loathe; the aroma can be overpowering if the oil is used neat on the skin. However, wheatgerm oil is an essential ingredient of facial massage mixtures (see page 101) and aromatherapy blends. Its high vitamin E content means that wheatgerm oil can be added to massage oils or skin creams as a natural preservative because the vitamin E acts as a powerful anti-oxidant and prevents the oil from becoming rancid. It is a good idea to add a few drops of wheatgerm oil to any massage oil that is kept in a warm, light environment such as the bathroom. Wheatgerm oil is added in this way to some capsule supplements to prolong their shelf-life, and a few drops shaken into a bottle of cooking oil is also an effective way of delaying oxidation and rancidity.

4

The Skin in the Sun

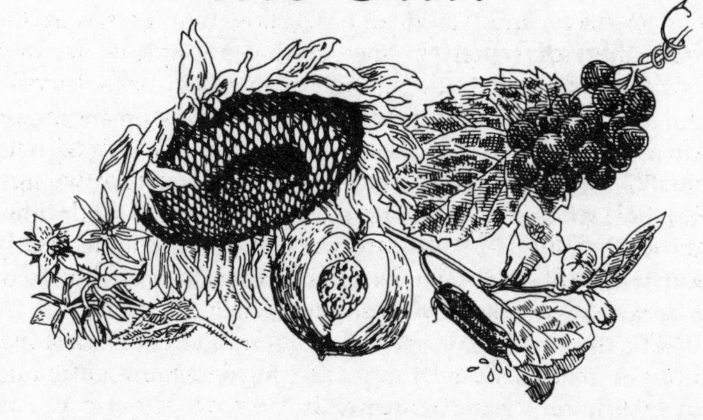

In addition to repairing the skin from within as well as from the outside, there is one other important part of skincare that will save your skin from the signs of growing old. Protecting the skin from the sun is the most effective way of warding off wrinkles, and dermatologists the world over have described sunblock as being the only anti-ageing cream that really works. In 1980, the Chief Dermatologist of Massachusetts General Hospital, Dr Thomas Fitzpatrick, announced to the medical world that 'sun is one of the four deadly pleasures of life, the others being alcohol, nicotine and food'. As this senior skin specialist states, these can all be extremely damaging to the skin.

The knowledge that strong sunshine destroys the skin is nothing new and has been an accepted fact for a decade or more. The sales of sunscreen during the summer months have soared over the last few years and most of us now pack a sunblock into our holiday suitcase. What is increasingly worrying, however, is that all new research into the relationship between the sun and skin states that the sun's rays are the number one cause of all facial lines, skin sagging and premature skin ageing. Even the feeble British sunshine that creeps through the clouds on an overcast day can cause chaos beneath the surface of the skin. It is clear that the only way we will win the war on wrinkles is with a two-tiered approach. Firstly, the internal use of vital oils to repair the skin, and secondly, the external use of a skincare regime that includes sunscreens to shield the surface of the face.

Sun-Worshipping

Idolising the sun is not a modern-day phenomenon and dates back to many ancient civilisations. As long ago as 2000BC, Egyptian kings were crowned as sons of the sun-god, Re, and built temples and shrines to honour him. Across the globe in South America, the ancient Aztec tribes also worshipped the sun and constructed golden palaces and monuments decorated with images of the sunflower. By 135AD, the Greek physician, Anthyllos, had concluded that sunlight made people stronger and fitter, although it would take much longer to discover why.

In addition to sustaining all forms of life on this planet, the sun has two direct actions on the human body. Being in strong sunlight stimulates the pituitary gland; this master endocrine gland at the base of the brain controls hormone secretions and regulates our moods and emotions. It is a fact of life that we feel happier in warmer weather as the bright sunshine encourages the pituitary gland to send cheery signals to the brain. It is also no coincidence that countries with low levels of natural daylight, such as Scandinavia during the winter months, have the highest rates of depression and suicide. There is even a medically recognised mental illness thought to be caused by low sunlight levels. Known as Seasonal Affective Disorder (SAD), this extreme form of winter blues can be treated effectively with a long holiday in the sun or a course of bright-light therapy. Unfortunately, only the latter option is available on the National Health Service.

In addition to being of psychological benefit, the sun also acts on the body by stimulating the supply of vitamin D through the skin. This is the only vitamin that the body can manufacture and proves that mankind was definitely designed to spend some time outdoors. However, we do not need strong sunlight to synthesise vitamin D and as long as some part of your body sees daylight regularly you will not fall deficient. Vitamin D has recently been cited as a potential cancer preventer, especially for breast and colon cancer. This has lead to articles being written about sunshine being good for the body and a positive health benefit. While a moderate amount of sun will increse your vitamin D levels, this should not be taken as an excuse to deep-fry the skin. Excessive sun exposure can *cause* some cancers as easily as low levels may be able to prevent it, and a safer option is to obtain your vitamin D through a source such as cod liver oil. American dermatologist, Neslon Lee Novick, believes that the vitamin D issue has been overplayed and says 'all the sun-induced vitamin D synthesis that you need can be had from one fifteen-minute period of sun exposure to an area of your skin no larger than the back of your hand'. Beyond that daily level, anything else is likely to hurt, not help, the skin. Those who may be at risk from vitamin D deficiency, however, are the housebound and Asian girls who are covered completely from head to toe when outdoors. Both these groups would do well to take a daily dose of cod liver oil which is naturally high in vitamin D.

Ban the Tan

Despite mankind's early worship of the sun, the fashion for acquiring a sun-tan is a relatively new skin craze. Until Victorian and early Edwardian times, pale skin was considered the most fashionable, and the only people to be seen with tans were peasants and labourers. A fair complexion was a sign of noble birth and society ladies went to extreme lengths to preserve their skins beneath huge hats, veils and parasols. No one dreamt of deliberately damaging the skin by exposing it to the sun.

All this changed in the early 1930s when the clothes designer, Coco Chanel, returned from a summer cruise with the Duke of Westminster (her lover at the time) shamelessly sporting a dark brown sun-tan. Suddenly the trend for a golden glow caught on and Mademoiselle Chanel set the upper-classes scurrying to fry themselves in the South of

France. A sun-tan was seen as a sign that you were either wealthy enough to take exotic holidays or so laid-back that you spent most of your time lazing outdoors. The trend for tanned skin peaked in the late 1960s when Brigitte Bardot joined the smart set in St. Tropez for a spot of serious sun-worshipping. Today, a quick glance at the actress's heavily-lined complexion says more about the effects of sun-bathing than words alone. Fortunately, the tide of public opinion has turned once more and it is thankfully no longer fashionable to burn the palest complexion to a dark shade of shoe leather.

The danger signs

A sun-tanned skin is a damaged skin and you can easily measure the amount of damage done to your skin just by the depth of your tan. There is no such thing as developing a 'safe tan'; it simply does not exist. As Dr John Hawk (head of the photobiology unit at St. Thomas' Hospital, London) states, 'the only safe tan is the one you were born with'. Those who are born with naturally fair skin are unfortunately most at risk from sun damage. This is because their skins contain low levels of the natural pigment melanin that protects the skin. Those with olive or light brown skins have about five times as much natural protection from the sun due to their higher quantities of melanin pigment, while those with black skin have ten to fifteen times the in-built protection. This genetic programming of the skin is nature's way of safeguarding the complexions of those native to hotter climates such as the Middle East and Africa. However, even black skin, despite its high levels of melanin, is prone to sun-induced skin-ageing and no matter what colour your complexion is, we are all at risk from the sun's rays.

A sun-tan is a warning that your skin is in danger. It develops when the melanocyte cells in the epidermis that contain the pigment melanin are activated by ultra-violet light from the sun. Sunlight is pure energy and consists of infra-red rays of heat which we feel, visible light which we can see (that is the colour spectrum of red, orange, yellow, green, blue, indigo and violet) and ultra-violet or invisible light. These rays travel to earth in a combination of waves of different dimensions, zigzagging through space into our atmosphere. It is the invisible ultra-violet light which ultimately penetrates the skin that is the most dangerous for our complexion. Ultra-violet light is divided into three groups:

UVA

The first is ultra-violet A (UVA) which has the longest wavelength of 320–400 nanometres. These represent 80 per cent of all the ultra-violet radiation that reaches the earth from the sun. UVA rays not only hit the surface of the skin but they also pass straight through it and reach the depths of the dermis below. UVA rays trigger a range of sun-induced allergies and increase the cancer-causing effects of UVB (see below). UVA rays also destroy collagen and elastin fibres and generate free-radicals within the skin. UVA radiation is recognised as one of the most significant factors in skin ageing.

UVB

The second group is ultra-violet B (UVB) with a medium wavelength of 290-320 nanometres. UVB rays represent 20 per cent of all ultra-violet radiation but are much more energetic than UVA and cause serious skin damage. UVB rays are absorbed mainly in the epidermis and upper layers of the dermis and stimulate the production of the pigment melanin which gives us our tan. UVB rays also help with the synthesis of vitamin D. Too much UVB radiation causes erythema or reddening of the skin and sunburn. UVB rays are also mostly responsible for causing skin cancers.

UVC

The third group is ultra-violet C (UVC) which has the shortest wavelength of 200–290 nanomentres. UVC emits the highest form of radiation and, if allowed to reach the earth, would totally destroy all living cells on the planet; life as we know it would cease to exist. Fortunately, UVC is blocked by the earth's ozone layer and does not reach us – yet.

It is easy to remember the effects of ultra-violet radiation on the skin: UVA rays cause the most AGEING while the UVB rays are responsible for BURNING.

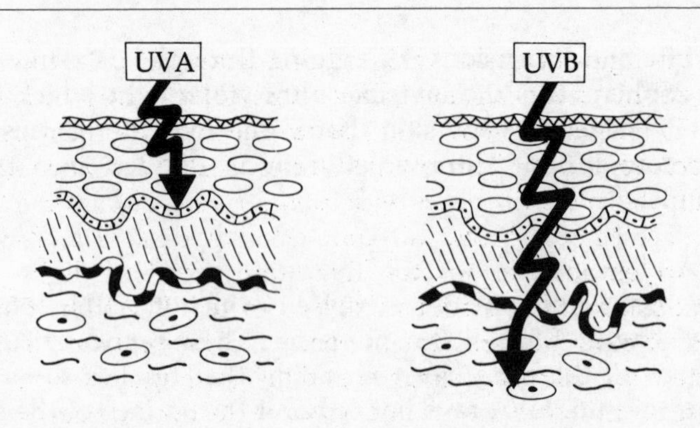

Dying for a tan?

We expose our skin to ultra-violet radiation each time we step outside the front door. A scorching summer day is clearly more dangerous than a rainy one, but even a bright wintry morning can signal damage occurring deep in the depths of the skin.

The main health risk with all sun-bathing is the increased risk of skin cancer. The good news is that skin cancer is *always* curable provided it is caught early enough. If left too late, however, malignant melanomas will kill. Despite being the only form of cancer to be 100 per cent curable, the rate of skin cancer is increasing at an alarming rate (the fastest increase of any type of cancer) and this is directly due to our sun exposure. Over one thousand people die needlessly from malignant melanoma every year in Britain alone, and this statistic is rising fast.

The dramatic increase in skin cancers in recent years is largely due to the fairer-skinned taking more holidays in tropical climates and not protecting their skins. While this is worrying, it is at least easy to remedy by promoting the use of sunblocks, protective hats and clothing. A more frightening risk factor is the thinning ozone layer that is gradually reducing and allowing more of the sun's powerful rays to penetrate than ever before. An unpublished United Nations study has predicted that the incidence of skin cancers and cataracts will continue worldwide due to the continuing thinning of the ozone layer. According to the UN scientific review, cases of skin cancer will show an annual *increase* of 300,000, and eye cataracts will increase by 1.75 million worldwide if reduction of the ozone layer by 10 per cent occurs and persists. While the thinning ozone layer no longer hits the headlines, a new study by the Department of the Environment shows that the ozone layer has been cut by 8 per cent over Europe alone and that our ozone cover could be reduced by as much as 30 per cent by the year 2000. It is not only the fair-skinned who are at risk. The UN report emphasises for the first time that both light- and dark-skinned populations will be affected. In addition to the risk of skin cancers, the increase in UV radiation is predicted to trigger damage to the immune system and increase the incidence or severity of infectious diseases.

The Australians have acknowledged the danger of the sun for several years and have developed much greater public awareness than other countries. This is largely because the first hole in the ozone layer occurred directly above Australia, leading to vastly increased cases of fatal skin cancers. Today, the message from the Australian Government Health Department is simple and to the point: posters urging you to 'slip, slop, slap' are seen all over Australia and are translated as meaning slip on a shirt, slop on a sunscreen and slap on a hat. Australians adore the great outdoors, but if you visit the country today you will notice that their skins have become visibly paler over the last few years. You will also see many health education posters explaining how to spot a skin cancer before it develops beyond the treatable stage.

The cancer connection

The commonest kind of skin cancer is *solar keratosis*. It looks like rough, reddish-brown patches of skin and is found on the least protected parts of the body, such as the face, hands and arms. These patches are easily removed by freezing but tend to reappear in sunlight so sufferers must stay in the shade. Basal cell cancers, sometimes called rodent ulcers, are small fleshy bumps that commonly appear on the side of the nose. These are unique in the cancer world because they are always completely curable. However, squamous cell cancers are faster-growing lumps and are a more dangerous breed of skin sore. The most sinister of all, however, is the malignant melanoma which kills hundreds of thousands of people each year worldwide. Even this most deadly skin disorder can be treated successfully if it's caught quickly.

For some unknown reason, malignant melanomas are more common in women than men and mostly affect the fair-skinned. What we do know is that skin cancer often occurs some years after severe sunburn due to over-exposure to the sun's UVB radiation. The first symptom is usually a mole which starts to itch, followed by other rapid changes in its shape, size and colour. Be especially aware of a mole with an irregular outline or one which becomes inflamed or bleeds. The earlier malignant melanomas are detected, the easier they are to treat, so if you are at all suspicious about your skin consult your GP without delay. It also pays to check your family's skin regularly, and men must watch out for unusual moles on the head – especially if they have a bald patch or their hair is thinning.

The danger of the sun cannot be over-emphasised and just one incidence of severe sunburn in childhood more than doubles the risk of developing skin cancer in later life. All children need to be protected from the sun during the summer months, especially if they play outdoors in strong sunshine. Try to cover them up as much as possible but be aware that cotton fabrics only block about 50 per cent of all UVB radiation. Wide-brimmed hats are useful, as are total sunblocks (buy waterproof brands if the child is going into the sea or swimming pool).

While the best form of protection comes from covering up the skin, there is also an internal precaution that everyone can take. The vitamin beta carotene (the vegetable precursor to vitamin A) has been found to reduce the effects of sun damage on the skin and appears to have quite a strong anti-cancer action. According to John Dickinson, professor of nutrition at Surrey university, a daily dose of beta carotene makes the body more resistant to sun damage and can help the body fight the sun's rays from within. While this should not be used as the only method of sun protection, it is probably worth taking extra beta carotene for a few weeks before going on holiday or during an exceptionally warm British summer. Beta carotene can be taken in capsule form or obtained by eating plenty of carrots, parsley, spinach, sweet potatoes (yams), broccoli and cantaloupe melons.

Sun-induced Ageing

It's not just our health that is at stake here for the sun is also the number one cause of premature ageing. Skin scientists have estimated that the sun's rays cause 99 per cent of all premature wrinkles, while the effects of gravity account for just 1 per cent.

While UVB radiation can quickly burn unprotected skin and increase the risk of developing skin cancer, it also encourages freckling, uneven pigmentation and 'liver spots' on the backs of the hands. These particular blemishes have nothing to do with the liver and are officially called lentigines. They are sun-induced, over-pigmented freckles with distinct, irregular borders. They commonly occur on the backs of the hands as this is the one area of the body that is rarely covered up or protected by a sunblock. Liver spots can start appearing as early as age 30 and once they are with you they will not disappear. Bleaching creams are not very effective and can irritate the skin and cause uneven blotchiness. The only permanent removal of liver spots is to have them burned off with low pulses of electricity (electrodesiccation), removed with chemical skin peeling agents or frozen off with liquid nitrogen (cryotherapy). Laser treatment may also work for some and is less painful. Another option is to conceal the marks with a waterproof camouflage cream. Of course, prevention is always far easier than cure.

Factors in our diet may play a part in the formation of pigmentation marks and an American study into the use of anti-oxidant nutrients has revealed some interesting findings. In a study of 200 elderly testers, 100 were given a daily dose of vitamin E and other anti-oxidants while the remainder were supplied with a placebo. At the end of a 12-month period, those who had been given the real supplements had fewer patches of increased pigmentation and less liver spots than those given the dummy capsules.

UVA and the free radical factor

The damage caused by UVA is even more invidious as it does not show up on the surface of the skin but occurs deep in the depths of the dermis. UVA rays are recognised by dermatologists as playing a bigger role than UVB in skin ageing. They gradually destroy the firm texture of collagen and elastin fibres, causing the skin to thicken and lose its natural elasticity and develop irreversible wrinkles.

UVA radiation is responsible for an approximate annual loss of 1 per cent of all collagen supplies in older skin. As women have slightly less collagen than men to start with, our faces are the first to fall. UVA radiation is also the principle cause of free radical damage beneath the surface of the skin and is increasingly recognised by cosmetic companies as the number one skincare problem. According to Dr Daniel Maes, head of scientific research at the Estée Lauder group, 'the free-radicals produced by ultra-violet light are particularly potent – it's a chain reaction, with one free-radical generating thousands more, similar to a nuclear reaction inside an atom bomb'. The explosive effect within the skin occurs beneath the surface, where the eye cannot see what is happening, and by the time the wrinkles have appeared on the face it is largely too late. As Dr Maes candidly admits '*nothing* can repair the damage already done and the emphasis must always be on prevention'.

The anti-ageing anti-oxidants

Fortunately for the face, there are powerful weapons that fight free-radical activity within the skin as soon as it starts. They are called anti-oxidants and, as we have seen (page 14), they are beta carotene, vitamin C (ascorbic acid) or vitamin E (d-alpha-tocopherol). The best sources of these nutrients are in plants, where the anti-oxidants are found in darker pigments produced by the plant's chlorophyll. A plant's level of anti-oxidants can have a quite spectacular effect on its existence. One of the oldest recorded plants still in existence is the chapparall bush from southern USA. This shrub is over 14,000 years old and 60 per cent of its dry weight consists of anti-oxidant nutrients – this is the secret of its outstanding longevity.

The same vitamins can help us to preserve our complexions and save our skin from the ageing effects of the sun. They are all important nutrients which we should be taking daily in our diet, not only for good health but also for the sake of our skin. While it is unrealistic even to try to turn back the in-built chronological clock that naturally ages the skin, there is a great deal that we can do to minimise the damage.

Premature ageing is often referred to by skin specialists as 'photo-ageing' and this is perfectly preventable by controlling free radical activity within the skin. Most visible signs of ageing are caused by UV light breaking down the collagen and elastin fibres in the dermis and increasing harmful enzyme activity within the skin. The collagenase enzyme destroys collagen while the elastase enzyme wipes out elastin, and both are triggered by exposure to UV light. Vitamin E and beta carotene help mop up most of the free-radical activity linked to such destruction, and vitamin C is also essential for controlling the activity of collagenase and for instructing the fibroblast cells to produce more collagen.

Anti-oxidant nutrients have been adopted by the cosmetics world for some time and they are amongst the more useful ingredients in skin creams and suncare products. Various versions of vitamin A are included in many moisturisers and vitamin E cream is a time-tested favourite. Even vitamin C, a very active molecule which needs to be kept isolated from other substances to prevent it inter-reacting and breaking down, can now be encapsulated and added to skin creams. Of course, the anti-oxidants are most effective when supplied internally and are an important part of our skincare diet. Some nutritionists believe that early man was able to produce his own anti-oxidant nutrients in the body (as we do vitamin D), but lost this talent through evolution. Some animals retain this ability and rats can make vast quantities of vitamin C, equivalent to producing 10,000 mg each day in humans.

Sun Repair and Vitamin E

As well as preventing the very visible signs of premature ageing, vitamin E is especially useful when it comes to repairing severely sun-damaged or even burnt skin. Vitamin E is the most effective quencher of UV-induced free radical activity and dramatically reduces skin damage. It is also a well-documented healer, and sunburn in particular responds well to vitamin E ointment or natural wheatgerm oil.

In his book *The Vitality Vitamin*, Dr Len Mervyn reports the extraordinary case of a girl suffering from intense sunburn over most of her body who was liberally covered with vitamin E ointment. After an hour of her treatment she recovered completely, with no signs of blisters or peeling. Another case reported that a man, with bad sunburn on his back, applied the same treatment, but could only reach half his back. The following day there was no sign of sunburn on skin treated with vitamin E, but the other half of his back was covered in large blisters. Photographs of this case were taken and used to present the case for vitamin E used topically (on the skin) to a medical congress in California.

Serious burns and scalds are obviously more damaging than sunburn, but vitamin E is also an effective treatment. Applications of vitamin E in a daily dose of 300 iu have proved proficient in cases of severe burns. The healing properties of vitamin E on the skin have been attributed to reducing the pain shortly after application, preventing the burn from deepening by limiting cell damage and stimulating the rapid regeneration of new skin. Vitamin E is one of the most important ingredients to look for in an after-sun product and it is worth taking a bottle of wheatgerm oil with you on holiday in case of accidental sunburn.

Sensible Suncare

Despite the enormous amount of damage the sun does to the skin, we do not have to shroud ourselves from head to toe before setting foot outside. When it comes to ageing, the main concern for all of us is with our face and this is the most important area to be protected. Personally, I use a high-factor sunscreen on my face and neck every day, either one that has been incorporated into a moisturiser or foundation, or a separate sunblock if I am going into strong sunlight. Having been a serious sun-worshipper in my teens (spending a scorching New York summer roasting on the roof of a Manhattan skyscraper with little more than a dab of baby lotion for 'protection'), I already have my share of wrinkles for later life, but my no-tan face plan will at least minimise the damage of wayward youth. When it comes to the rest of the body, I use a moderate form of sun protection as I do not really mind developing wrinkled arms or legs for the sake of the occasional golden glow. However, my face will always be protected in the years to come and given the best possible chance of survival.

Brownie points

When buying a sunscreen, the way to choose your level of protection is to look at the Sun Protection Factor (SPF) given on the side of the bottle. The higher the number, the greater the degree of protection. The SPF was introduced to give guidance as to how long you could stay in the sun before becoming sunburnt. A product marked SPF 8 will, theoretically, allow you to stay out eight times longer than if you were not wearing any protection. The amount of protection you need depends principally on your natural skin colouring; the paler your skin, the greater the defence required. If a moisturiser states that it contains a sunscreen, make sure you know what SPF it is, as it is often too low to be of much benefit. However, you could build up your protection by using a moisturiser with, say, an SPF 6 together with a foundation that has an SPF 4 to give you a total protection factor of 10. Adding a further layer of face powder would also increase your resistance to UV light as all make-up contains powdered particles that help block out the sun's rays. It must be noted, however, that most SPF numbers apply only to the level of protection given against UVB radiation, and the amount of protection from UVA rays is often a good deal less. Always check on the package to ensure your skin will be guarded against both UVA and UVB radiation.

Message in a bottle

The first sunscreens were developed during World War I for fighter pilots to protect their faces in their open-topped cockpits. The thick zinc oxide paste they were given was effective but messy and turned the skin a ghoulish white. Other early formulations included an old Tibetan recipe containing 5 per cent tannic acid which was successfully used on the skin of mountaineers, the only snag being that it corroded their iron climbing equipment. During World

War II, chemical sunscreens were developed to protect troops fighting in tropical countries. Shortly after the end of the War, one of the first suncare ranges, Coppertone, was created by a Miami Beach pharmacist who noticed that tourists relied on ineffective home-made concoctions. Since then, sunscreen ingredients have become increasingly sophisticated and while some of the original ingredients, such as zinc oxide, remain, manufacturing techniques have improved and products are much more pleasant to use.

Powdered minerals, such as zinc oxide, ferric oxide and titanium dioxide, work by providing a physical barrier on the skin that reflects or scatters the sun's rays. These are highly effective at blocking both UVA and UVB radiation and are the safest ingredients to use on a sensitive skin. The drawback in the past with these powdered mineral filters was that they tended to leave a white sheen on the skin and could not be formulated into high-tec suncare sprays, gels and oils. Recent advances in cosmetic technology, however, have led to titanium dioxide being micronised into particles that are 20 times smaller than previously possible, making them appear transparent on the skin. This process of micronisation also makes the mineral more versatile and it can now be found in a wide range of suncare and cosmetic preparations.

The other group of sunscreen ingredients are the chemical filters that react with the skin to prevent the UV rays from reaching the lower levels of the skin. The disadvantage of chemical sunfilters is that you need a high level of chemicals to block out most of the sun's rays and this can lead to irritation of the skin. Chemical sunscreens are also not as efficient as the powdered minerals at blocking harmful UVA radiation. They work by absorbing the UV radiation and preventing it from passing through the skin. The chemicals commonly found in sunscreens include PABA (the B-vitamin para-aminobenzoic acid) which was considered one of the most effective sunscreens a decade ago. However, it does not absorb as much UVB as the newer chemical derivatives, stains clothing and can irritate the skin. Other UVB sunscreens include Padimate O (a PABA derivative) which is water resistant, cinnamates (found to be gentler on the skin), homosalate and octyl salicylate. There are few effective chemical UVA sunscreens, such as benzophenone

3, which are able to protect the skin against the ageing effects of UVA as well as the burning of UVB. It is well worth reading the ingredient listing on the back of the bottle of sunscreen to see exactly which type of protection it offers.

Natural plant oils also offer some natural protection as they screen out some of the sun's harmful rays. Sesame oil, for example, blocks nearly a third of all UVA and UVB radiation and is often added to sun oils and lotions for its skin-softening properties. As an emergency measure, sesame oil can be used on its own if you run out of sunscreen, but in these days of the thinning ozone layer it is not strong enough to be your sole source of sun protection. Your best option in terms of maximum UVA and UVB protection with minimum risk of irritation is to choose a sunscreen with a high level of powdered or micronised minerals and skin-softening natural oils.

Sunscreen ingredients

UVA	*UVB*
Benzophenone 3	PABA
Octyl Methoxycinnamate	Octyl Methoxycinnamate
Octyl Salicylate	Octyl Salicylate
Octocrylene	Homosalate

Some brands also include useful cocktails of free-radical scavengers including vitamins A and E and even a synthetic form of the skin's own melanin, which offers the skin additional safeguards.

Anti-wrinkle face creams

The only effective anti-ageing cream is a sunblock. When choosing your level of facial protection, follow these wrinkle-free guidelines:

Pale skins – not less than SPF 15 daily. Total sunblock when in strong sunshine.
Medium skins – not less than SPF 12 daily. Total sunblock when in strong sunshine.
Dark skins – not less than SPF 8 daily and SPF 15 when in strong sunshine.

Please note: There is absolutely no point in spending any money at all on expensive anti-ageing creams unless you use a high-factor sunscreen. It's like joining Weight Watchers while eating 10 boxes of chocolates a day – there is no way a moisturiser can ever improve the effects of the sun on unprotected skin.

The holiday sun-tan

Although the trend for an unnaturally dark tan is fading fast, most pale-skinned people still aspire to a 'healthy looking' golden glow. For those who still want to get their bodies lightly browned (never the face), here is your checklist for holiday tanning:

- the higher the SPF number on a suncare product, the greater the protection for your skin
- always use a high-factor sunscreen (SPF 15 or above) for the first few days of sunbathing in a hot climate. This gives your body a chance to acclimatise
- apply your sunscreen before you leave your room, not while sitting on the beach. Allow it to sink into the skin before dressing or you may wipe some off
- re-apply sunscreen to all areas of exposed skin every few hours. Use a waterproof formula when swimming and re-apply after towelling dry
- the sun's rays penetrate the ozone layer so have no difficulty cutting through the clouds. Use a sunscreen even on a cloudy day
- sunscreens are not just for sun-bathing but should also be used when sightseeing, eating on the terrace or playing sport outdoors
- always avoid the midday sun when UV radiation is strongest. One-third of the day's radiation is received between 10 a.m. and 2 p.m., when the sun is at its highest
- one way to tell when the sun is at its highest and most dangerous is to look at your shadow. If it is shorter than your actual height it means that the sun is up high and more likely to burn your skin
- never let the skin burn. Apart from causing serious skin damage and increasing your risk of skin cancer, this is also the fastest way to lose your tan

- be aware that UV light is reflected back from water such as the sea, lakes and swimming pools. It also reflects from snow which is why skiers and water-sports' enthusiasts alike need extra sun protection
- sensitive skin needs a total sunblock. Watch vulnerable areas such as ears, lips, scalp, breasts and nipples
- no matter what your skin colour, your face always needs a total sunblock to prevent premature ageing. Wear a hat to protect any areas you may have missed such as the scalp, neck and ears.

How to choose a sunscreen

Buying some form of suncare is essential if you want your body to develop a light brown tan while on holiday. This is easier said than done, as most chemists and department stores now have an enormous range to choose from. Ignore the glossy promotions and special offers and follow the simple suncare chart (overleaf) to find the products that offer you a safer tan. Remember, the more slowly you tan, the longer you will keep your colour. Do not be put off by higher SPF ratings or numbers – you will still develop a light tan but it may take a little longer than usual. Those holidaying in very hot, tropical climates should opt for the maximum protection.

Other factors that women should bear in mind when buying their suncare include what medication they are taking at the time. The contraceptive pill and hormone replacement therapy are the two main culprits for reacting with UVA and UVB rays to create a skin reaction called chloasma. Also known as 'pregnancy spots' or 'butterfly marks', these areas of blotchy, darkened skin pigmentation are linked to hormonal changes within the body and commonly appear on the cheeks, below the eyes and across the nose. As chloasma is triggered principally by strong UV light, those women at risk should seek the highest SPF indices when choosing suncreams for their faces. Unfortunately, chloasma marks are irreversible and the only option once they have developed is to cover them with a concealing cream. It is also worth buying enough suncare to last throughout your holiday as the very high factors may not be available at your destination. Bear in mind that all sun-tanned skin is damaged skin; it is simply a question of degree.

type of skin	*recommended SPF range*
Never tans, always burns	15+ or total sunblock
Tans eventually, but burns easily	10–15+
Tans easily, burns occasionally	6–12+
Always tans, rarely burns	4–8+

Children in the sun

Children are a special group as they have thinner skins than adults and require greater levels of protection. Babies under 12 months of age cannot produce enough melanin to give their skin any natural protection at all, and fair-skinned babies must be kept out of the sun altogether. During the summer months it is essential that you fit a parasol or sunshade to the pram and head for the shady areas in the park or garden.

Once mobile, children are not so easy to control and toddlers need optimum protection such as loose cotton clothing and a hat. In Australia, nursery school children are kitted out with compulsory wide-brimmed hats which must be worn in the playground. It takes between 12 and 24 hours for sunburn to reach its greatest intensity, so bring a child in from the sun at the first sign of pink skin. Be aware that the sun's rays can penetrate clouds, so even on relatively dull days children need to be adequately protected. On sunnier days, children who are playing outdoors can even burn in the shade because UV light is scattered and reflected by surfaces such as sand, concrete and even grass. Always use a waterproof sunblock on children who are playing in the sea or swimming pool and re-apply after towelling them dry. Some brands of sunscreen are available as handy sprays and a quick squirt is the easiest way to top up a wriggling child's protection.

Try to keep children in the shade between the hours of 11 a.m. and 1 p.m. when the sun is at its fiercest, and make sure children drink plenty of water or diluted fruit juice to prevent dehydration. Most importantly, never, ever underestimate the strength of the sun. Childhood sun-exposure is thought to lead to 70 per cent of all skin slackening in adulthood but it is not just a question of warding off premature wrinkles (although the renowned American dermatologist, professor Albert Kligman, does suggest using a sunscreen *daily* from an early age). As we have seen, a single case of severe sunburn more than doubles your child's risk of skin cancer in later life. The answer is to protect and survive.

The Sunbed Story

As the sun is so damaging to the body, are sunbeds the answer for a safe tan? Unfortunately the answer is no, although they are certainly much safer than they used to be. When first introduced in the 1970s, sunbeds were made with tubes that emitted both UVA and UVB radiation. It soon became clear that the UVB radiation was actually burning the skin and these tubes were phased out. Virtually all sunbeds now rely on 'safer' UVA radiation. While UVA is unlikely to burn the skin and probably won't cause cancer on its own, it does penetrate deep into the dermis and damages the supporting structure of the skin. If you want to preserve your skin, do not use a sunbed. I have a cynical view of beauty salons that firstly encourage their clients to use increasingly high-pressured sunbeds and then recommend expensive anti-ageing facials. A far better option would be to ditch the sunbeds and start offering some serious skincare advice.

Faking it

Finally, the news we have all been waiting for. Yes, there *is* a way you can get a *safe* tan after all; it's called a *fake* tan. The tan that comes out of a bottle is the only one that will not damage the skin or lead to premature ageing. If the last time you tried a fake tan your legs looked as if they had been dipped in gravy browning, relax, formulations have moved on since then. Although the fake tans contain the same basic tanning agent, their textures and performance have vastly improved over the last couple of years. All fake tans work by permanently staining the uppermost hardened skin cells with a mineral salt called dihydroxyacetone. This develops on the skin into a fairly natural-looking shade of brown which lasts until the skin cells drop off. On average, a fake tan will last about 4–6 days, depending on your rate of cellular turnover. It is the dihydroxyacetone that gives all fake tanning creams a faintly yeasty smell, although most new formulations are able to mask this with other fragrances (it is worth sniffing them before you buy).

This type of self-tan does not wash off, so it is important to get it right when putting it on to the skin. If you follow these golden rules you will get the best possible results. Firstly, always exfoliate the skin to remove flakes of dead skin cells before applying. You do not need to scrub the body hard; a swift rub-down with a flannel is sufficient to dislodge tiny clumps of skin cells. Next, apply a body lotion or body oil to thoroughly moisturise the skin (a few drops of johoba oil will lightly moisturise the body from head to toe). Allow the oil or body lotion to be thoroughly absorbed before using the fake tanning lotion. If you have not used a fake tan before, always do a patch-test at least 12 hours before applying it to the rest of the body. Choose an area on the inner arm and apply a tiny amount of the product. After a few hours you will be able to see if it has turned into a shade of brown that suits you and discover whether the formulation irritates your skin. When it comes to applying the fake tan to the rest of the body, you may find it easier to use a fine latex cosmetic sponge to ensure the cream goes on smoothly. Pay special attention to knees, ankles and elbows where excess cream can gather and will make the final result look patchy. Streakiness can be avoided by continually smoothing the cream into the skin using long, sweeping, upward strokes.

Always wash your hands immediately after applying a fake tan or you will end up with dark brown palms. If you want naturally brown-looking hands, squeeze a small amount of cream on to the back of one hand and use it to rub across the back of the other hand. Many brands now offer fake tans in a choice of shades; if in doubt, experiment with the one nearest to your own skin colouring first. Fake tans may be used successfully on the face, although they tend to look blotchy if your face has any dry or flaky areas. A less permanent answer are wash-off facial tans, bronzing creams, gels and powders which all give the illusion of sun-kissed skin without the harsh reality of its side-effects.

5

Facial Firmers

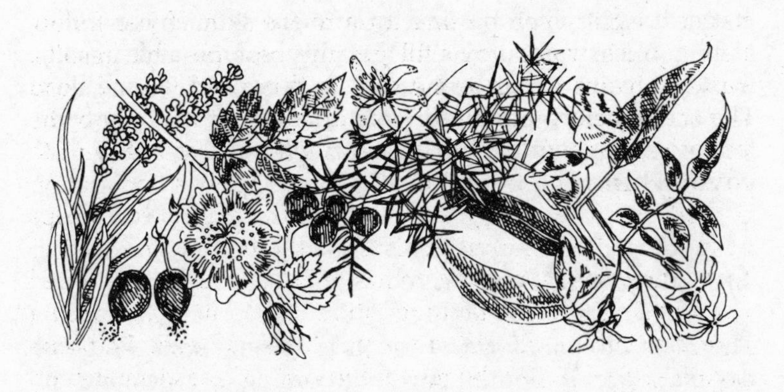

Strong, healthy skin can be kept in good shape with a few minutes of daily facial massage to strengthen and tone the skin. The act of massage has a powerful effect on our outer physique as well as our inner psyche by influencing the way we look and how we feel.

Massage relies purely on our sense of touch which is transmitted by a complicated network of nerve endings housed within the skin. When stimulated, these send messages of pleasure, relaxation or pain back to the brain. Our sense of touch is perhaps the most intimate and important of all our senses, yet it is also the most underrated. From mother and baby bonding to a more formal handshake or a comforting hug from a close friend, the act of touch has a powerful effect on biological processes in the body. Close body contact lowers our blood pressure and enables the blood supply to circulate more freely around the body. Psychologically, body contact is an important part of life and, although we tend to overlook it significance, it is a fundamental part of human behaviour.

Observations by the famous 'man-watcher', Dr Desmond Morris, have so far led to the naming of 457 different types of body contact, including specialist forms of touching by such people as doctors, dentists, priests and hairdressers.

The one area which seldom benefits from being touched however, is the face and neck. Dr Morris maintains that this is because we need to establish a strong bond of trust before we dodge away defensively when someone reaches for our face. Only the closest and oldest of friends, lovers, spouses or parents are allowed to put their hands on our faces. This instinctive fear is probably why so many women confess to feeling uneasy about visiting beauty salons and placing trust in a pair of unknown hands as they work on the skin. The act of touching our own skin, though, is not only comforting and soothing but also brings with it many real physical benefits.

The Magic of Massage

The most obvious form of touch is self-massage, and this has played an important part in grooming and cleaning rituals throughout the ages. From Swedish-style pummelling to relax knotted areas of tension in the shoulders, to the gentler and more intuitive art of aromatherapy, massage benefits the outer skin as well as the inner being.

All facial treatments carried out by professional beauty therapists incorporate a range of massage techniques, and facial massage is acknowledged to be one of the fastest ways to get the skin glowing. As soon as we start to massage the face or body we stimulate the circulation and bring fresh blood supplies to the surface of the skin. This replenishes the skin cells with many important nutrients and provides a welcome boost of oxygen, via the bloodstream, needed to sustain life within the cells.

Localised massage, such as the techniques that are described on page 89, also boost the lymphatic system responsible for clearing waste matter from skin cells. The lymphatic system consists of a network of channels that run parallel to blood vessels throughout the body. These channels are filled with a milky-white substance called lymph which acts as the body's dustman. The main function of lymph is to carry away the toxins and decomposing cellular material that clog the dermis and lead to a dull, devitalised complexion. Unlike our blood supply, however, lymph does not have a heart to pump it around the body and relies solely on exercise and external movement to stimulate its flow. By using a series of 'lymphatic drainage' massage techniques we can encourage the speedy elimination of waste matter which leads to a clearer, smoother complexion.

Sex and the Skin

There is no doubt that sex is good for the skin. The main reason for this is that close body contact releases surface tension in the skin and speeds the flow of blood to the erogenous zones (which include the face and neck). It goes without saying that the actual physical activity involved also boosts the overall blood circulation and lymphatic system. The energy expenditure involved in reaching orgasm is reported to be equivalent to taking a two-mile run and this level of physical activity is extremely healthy for the skin. Despite his wine and womanising, it is worth noting that Cassanova was also reputed to have a great complexion!

Emotional responses show up quickly on the face and it is no coincidence that those who are in love can be spotted simply by the radiant state of their skin. Blushing is also an excellent facial exercise and happens when the blood vessels in the dermis dilate to allow a surge of blood to the surface of the skin. However embarrassing at the time, those who flush easily benefit on each occasion from a fresh delivery of oxygen and nourishing nutrient supplies.

Facial Massage

Massage techniques for the face are both simple and effective. The only tools you need are a clean set of fingertips and a small amount of facial massage oil (see page 98). The rules for facial massage are straightforward: always work on freshly cleansed skin, do not touching weeping spots or active acne and never use more than the lightest, fingertip pressure. As we have seen, the skin is highly responsive to our sense of touch and the very gentlest movements are all that is needed to see a real improvement on the surface of the face.

Early morning massage

This routine is based on the principles of Do-In, a Japanese form of self-massage designed to re-balance the body and strengthen the skin from within. The entire routine takes about 15 minutes from start to finish; those with less time can choose the shorter version on page 93.

1. Sit in a comfortable position on the floor. Holding the palms of your hands against your cheeks, take three deep breaths in and out. Make sure you breathe in deeply through your nose, filling the diaphragm, and not the chest. This forces more oxygen into the lungs and enables the body to relax fully. Breathe out through your mouth, expelling all the air from the diaphragm with a loud sigh.
2. Rub the palms of your hands up and down your cheeks and the sides of your face until the skin becomes warm. This stimulates blood circulation and will get the skin glowing.
3. With thumbs resting beneath your jaw and using your fingertips only, lightly drum your fingers across your cheekbones and around your eyes in an anti-clockwise direction. Take your fingertips across your forehead and lightly tap over your forehead, around your temples and up into your hairline. Gently tug your hair near its roots, working from the front to the back of the head.

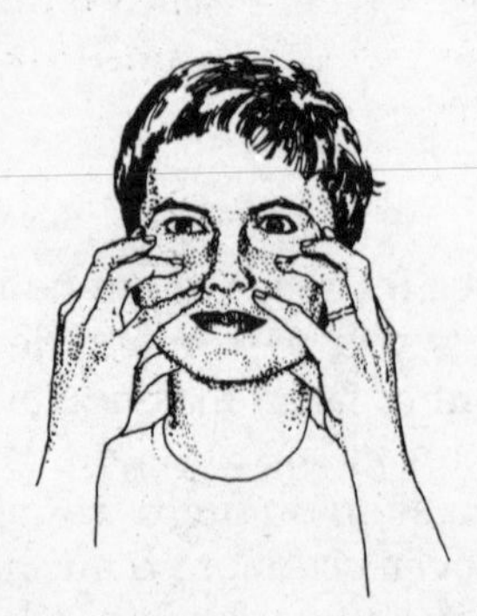

4. Using the tips of your index fingers, softly press the top of your nose just below where your eyebrows would normally meet. Stimulate this spot by gently circling your

fingertips for one minute. Still using the tips of your index fingers, trace a line from the top of your nose to the centre of your forehead. Repeat six times. The action of stimulating this area is important for energising the lymphatic system and helping to keep nasal and sinus passages clear.

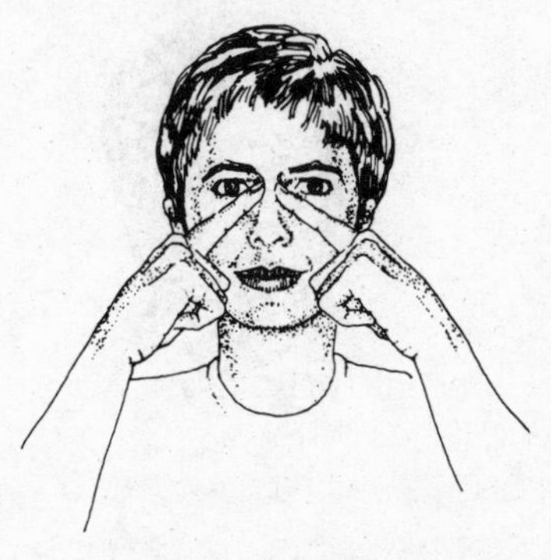

5 Close your eyes and place both palms over them. Relax the tension in your neck and feel the weight of your head being supported by your hands. Take three deep breaths in and out, filling and emptying the diaphragm as before.
6 With your eyes still closed, use the middle three finger tips to press lightly along the contours of the eye socket beneath the browbone. Repeat three times, working outwards. With your index fingers, lightly stroke the browbone just beneath the eyebrow, working from the inner eye outwards towards the temples. Repeat three times.

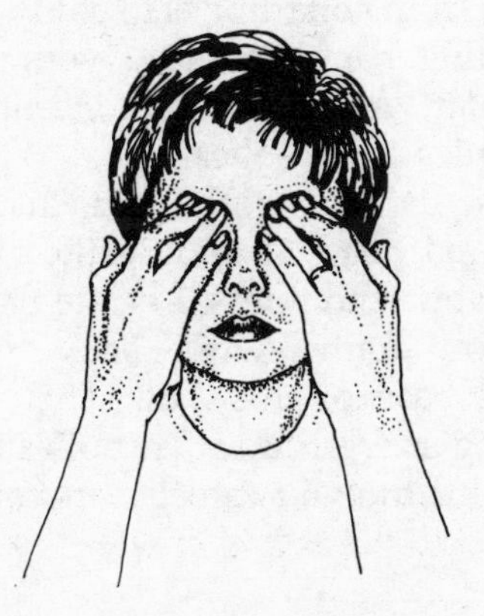

7 Using the ends of your index fingers, lightly press them against the sides of your nose and rub gently. This encourages blood and lymphatic circulation and helps to keep the skin either side of the nostrils free from spots and blackheads.

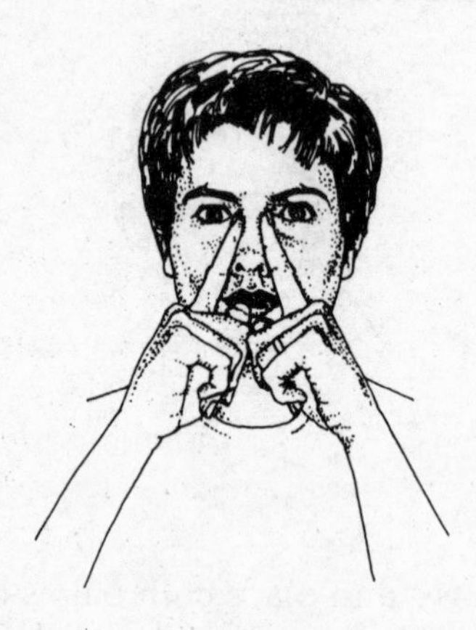

8 With your thumbs and forefingers, lightly pinch along your jawline from your chin to your ear lobes. Repeat the pinching movements, working back towards the centre of the chin.

9 Use your thumb and forefinger to squeeze your ear lobe and the outer edge of your ears lightly, from bottom to top.

10 Using the backs of your fingertips, lightly pat the skin under your chin and jawline. Finish by smoothing your neck with sweeping movements, using the backs of your hands, from collarbones to chin.

11 With firm fingertips, massage your entire face with small circular movements, concentrating on your cheeks, temples and forehead.

12 Make a loose fist with both hands and lightly tap your entire face and head, including the back of your neck and across your shoulders. Let the fists bounce off the scalp as you gently work back from the hairline towards the base of the skull. This action leaves the scalp tingling as fresh blood supplies rush to the skin's surface to feed the hair follicles and encourage healthy hair growth.

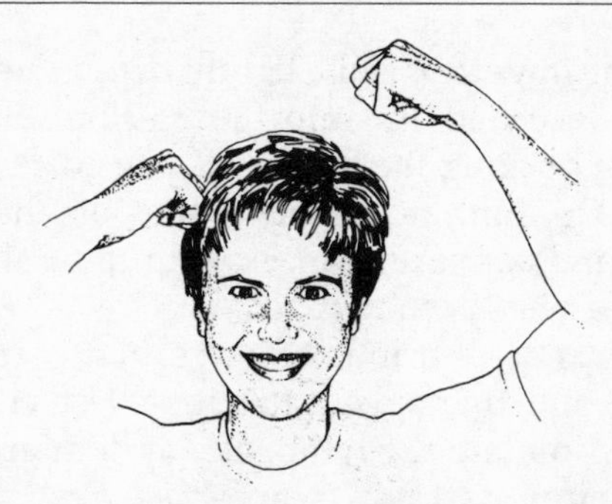

13 Tilt your head to one side until the right ear almost touches the right shoulder. Hold this position for 30 seconds before tilting your head to the other side. Hold this position for 30 seconds, then rotate your head until your chin touches your chest, then move your head slowly from side to side, stretching the muscles in your neck. Slowly tip your head backwards, pointing your chin towards the ceiling. While holding this position, open and close your mouth 10 times, feeling the muscles around your jaw tighten and relax. Finish by slowly circling your head twice to the right and twice to the left.

14 Finally, return to the starting position with both palms placed over your cheeks. Close your eyes and take three deep breaths in and out as before. Use this moment to visualise the air flowing freely throughout your body, energising every skin cell and helping your skin to grow smooth and strong.

Mini-morning massage

Those with one eye on breakfast and the other on the clock should not skip their early morning massage routine but can opt for this abridged version. It takes less than 5 minutes and once you have learnt the routine it can be done anywhere – in the bath, the shower or even while a passenger in the car.

1 Begin by placing your palms over your cheeks and taking three deep breaths, breathing in through your nose to swell the diaphragm, not the chest. Breathe out through your mouth, expelling all the air with a loud sigh.

2 Using your fingertips only, lightly drum the fingers over the neck, face and up into the hairline. Stimulate the scalp by massaging the head as if you were shampooing your hair. Concentrate on any tight spots that you feel in the scalp and continuing massaging until all the tension in your head has been released.
3 With the tips of your index fingers, gently rub the top of your nose on either side of the bone. Use circular movements to stimulate the lymphatic system and help keep nasal and sinus passages clear.
4 Using the tips of your index fingers, stroke the skin beneath your browbone, working from the inner corner of the eye out towards the temples. Repeat five times.
5 With the tips of your middle fingers, stroke the skin in a semi-circle from the inner eye down around the cheekbones, finishing with the fingertips at the top of the ear. Repeat five times.
6 Make a loose fist with both hands and lightly tap your face and head, including the back of your neck and across your shoulders. Let your fists bounce off your scalp as you work back from the hairline towards the base of the skull. This action leaves the scalp tingling as fresh blood supplies rush to the skin's surface to feed the hair follicles and encourage healthy hair growth.

The stress-buster

Nothing shows up faster on the face than the tension and stress that quickly build up during a busy working day. The muscles in our faces and necks can soon become hardened into a fixed, firm expression and, before we realise it, our brows have knotted together into an irreversible frown. If you feel the tension rising, take 5 minutes from your hectic schedule and de-stress the face with this simple routine. You do not even have to leave your chair, but the effect is the same as going to the beauty salon for a facial.

1 Relax your shoulders

Begin by relaxing the muscles in the shoulders that support the neck. Using your whole hand, gently squeeze each shoulder between your fingers and palm. Work from the outer edge of the shoulder in towards the neck, rotating the shoulder-blade and lifting each shoulder as you massage it to release the tension. Massage each shoulder in turn for one minute at a time, until the muscles in the shoulders and lower neck have fully relaxed.

2 Stretch your neck

Loosen your neck by gently rotating your head clockwise, using slow movements and never jerking or straining your throat. Repeat by circling your head anti-clockwise. Sit upright in the chair and hang your hand down until your chin rests lightly on your chest. Take three deep breaths in and out. Hang your head to the right until your right ear almost touches your right collarbone. Hold the stretch while taking three deep breaths in and out. Move your head to the back, tilting your chin until it points towards the ceiling. Take three deeps breaths in and out before circling your head around to the left. Hang your head in this final position until your left ear almost touches your left collarbone. Hold the stretch while taking three deep breaths in and out.

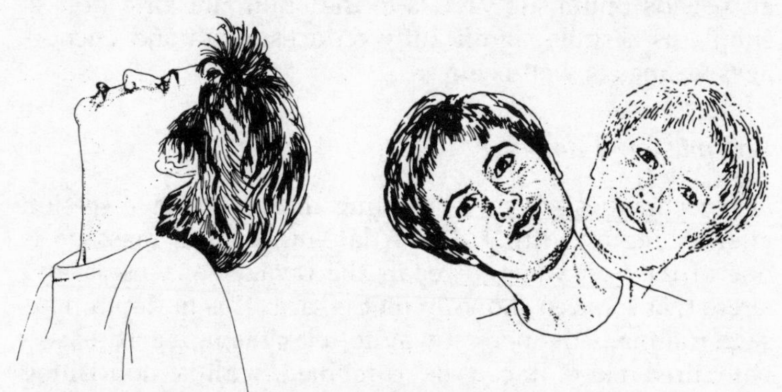

3 Wipe the tension from your face

With light, fingertip movements, gently tap the area around your eyes, working down across your cheeks and up into your temples and hairline. Use your knuckles to tap your forehead and scalp, finishing with a gentle pounding of the blood vessels and nerve endings located at the base of the skull.

4 Firm up the frown lines

Prevent occasional worry lines from turning into permanent wrinkles by smoothing out and stretching the skin. Wipe away frowns as they form by stroking your eyebrows and moving both brows up and down. Relax the rest of your face and your mouth by puffing out both cheeks. Move the trapped air around inside your mouth to stretch the skin from the inside.

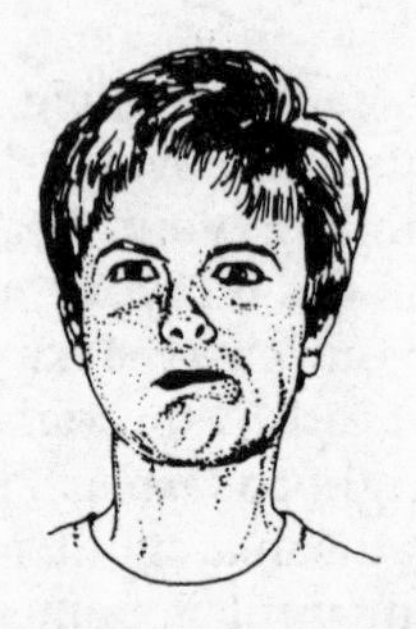

5 Say cheese!
Finish the stress-busting routine with a broad grin. Even if you do not feel like smiling, the action of pulling up the muscles tightens the supporting connective tissues. Smiling also sends optimistic signals to the brain and an action as simple as a smile significantly reduces stress and encourages feelings of well-being.

Bedtime wind-down

Few techniques are more relaxing than a massage session after a long and tiring day. A late-night facial massage is one of the best ways to repair the ravages of tension and stress that so often show up on the face. This in-depth massage routine is the perfect way to relax the face and rejuvenate tired skin. It can be combined with a nourishing massage oil for maximum benefit (see recipes on page 98). The bedtime wind-down routine is designed to be carried out on a regular basis, preferably at least once a week to see the best results. Long-distance travellers and those suffering from jet-lag will find that these techniques are a real boon for re-energising the skin and warding off signs of extreme fatigue.

1 Begin by pouring a small amount of massage oil into the palm of one hand. Rub your hands together to warm the oil before applying it to the surface of your skin. Using upward, sweeping movements, apply the massage oil from the base of your neck to the top of your forehead. If you do not mind getting your hair slightly oily, continue the movement right into the hairline and across the scalp.

2 Using your fingertips only, gently massage the skin in small circular movements, starting from the base of your neck and working upwards to your forehead. Concentrate on the jawline, cheeks and temples to stimulate the nerve endings and mobilise the lymphatic system.

3 With your fingertips held firmly together, press the skin along your hairline and across your entire forehead, working from the centre outwards with precise, firm movements. Press the skin along your browbones, just beneath each eyebrow, and finish by pressing along your jawline, working from the centre of the chin out towards the ears.

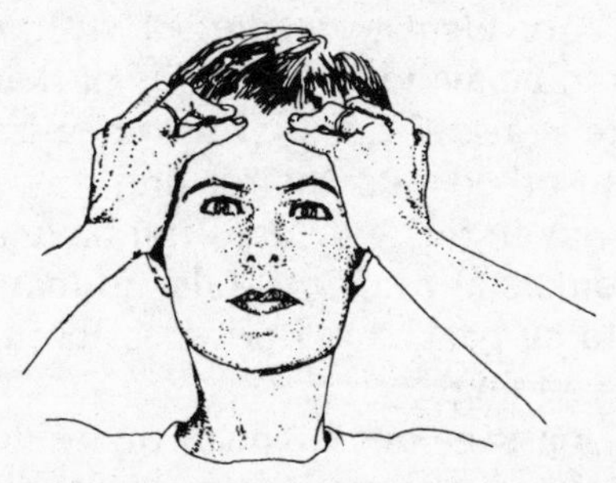

4 Using the tips of your index fingers, firmly stroke along each eyebrow six times, continuing the movement under your eyes so that you complete a circle around each eye socket. This action helps to decongest puffiness and will help reduce areas of swollen skin tissues surrounding your eyes.

5 Using the tips of your index fingers again, firmly stroke a curved line from the inner corner of your eye to your ear lobes, following the slope of the cheekbones. This line is a key part of the lymphatic system beneath the surface of the face and will help to keep the skin clear from within.

6 Using light patting movements, gently tap your entire face and neck working upwards from the collarbones.

This boosts fresh blood supplies to the surface of the skin and leaves the face and neck tingling. Having finished the massage routine, follow the energising facial exercises on page 103 to complete the treatment.

Facial Massage Oils

As well as nourishing the skin from within with oil supplements, vital oils can be used on the surface to smooth and soften. The best oils to use on the face and neck are enriched with natural vitamins, are light in texture but are non-greasy. As these oils are to be used directly on the face, it is well worth buying the best quality oils available, preferably cold-pressed or unrefined oils that are usually only on sale in specialised health shops. Never buy facial oils that are packaged in clear plastic bottles as these have been exposed to the light and may be rancid. Putting rancid oil directly on the skin is equivalent to feeding it with a dose of free radicals and is to be avoided. With oils packaged in plastic containers there is also the risk of the chemicals within the plastic being absorbed into the oil and any manufacturer that sells their oils in this way does not have the best interests of its customers at heart. All oils, no matter what their purpose, should be packed in dark glass bottles and stored away from heat and light.

Always buy massage oils in small quantities as they are very economical to use and a few drops go a long way. Buying in bulk is therefore a false economy as the oil is likely to have gone off before you reach the end of the bottle. Adding a few drops of wheatgerm oil to each bottle of massage oil will help prolong its shelf-life and boost the oil's vitamin E content, which in turn benefits the skin.

Almond oil

This slightly sticky oil is often used by aromatherapists as a base oil for massage as it provides a good 'slip' over the skin and does not sink in too quickly. Although useful for massage, some find it too greasy to use on the face and prefer to dilute it with a lighter oil. Unrefined almond oil is a useful source of vitamins and minerals and can also help to relieve the symptoms of itchy skin. The refined versions of almond oil sold by chemists do not contain high levels of nutrients but are useful as pure, hypo-allergenic moisturisers. Almond oil makes an excellent hand and nail cream and can also be added to the bath to relieve dry skin.

Apricot kernel oil

The light texture of this natural oil makes it a favourite for facial massage. Especially suited to dry, sensitive and more mature skins, apricot kernel oil is also a useful source of vitamins and contains traces of minerals. Unrefined versions of this oil contain small amounts of the free-radical-fighting anti-oxidant, vitamin E. As it is more expensive than other oils, apricot kernel oil may be mixed with a cheaper oil, such as almond or sunflower oil, for a less costly blend.

Avocado oil

This plant oil is a star performer in skincare. Easily absorbed by the skin, avocado oil is both revitalising and regenerating. Rich in vitamins and with traces of minerals, lecithin and essential fatty acids, this natural oil is an essential part of anti-ageing skincare. The best avocado oils are unrefined and still retain their sludgy green colour. They can be used neat on the face or body, added to the bath or blended with other oils to make facial massage blends.

Borage oil

This oil is not commonly available by the bottle and is most often found in capsule form. The easiest way to use this plant oil is to pierce a capsule with a pin and squeeze its contents into the palm of your hand. Very rich in the essential fatty acid GLA, borage oil is a useful addition to many massage oil blends. Borage oil can be used neat on dry, scaly skin or patches of atopic eczema. It is also especially helpful when treating dull, devitalised or heavily lined skin.

Evening primrose oil

This oil is also available in capsule form and can be used in the same way as borage oil. Evening primrose oil is also increasingly available in liquid form, either as a nutritional food supplement or as a massage oil. Because of its high levels of GLA, evening primrose oil is also useful when added to most facial oil blends, especially those designed to treat dry or mature complexions.

Grapeseed oil

Grapeseed oil is another favourite of aromatherapists as it is both lightweight and non-greasy. It can be used as a massage oil for both the face and body, but does not contain as many nourishing nutrients as other plant oils. Grapeseed oil is usually only available as a refined cooking oil but it is economical to use and appeals to some because of its lack of smell. It can be combined with other plant oils to boost its vitamin and mineral levels.

Hazelnut oil

This plant oil can be found in most supermarkets and is usually available in its natural, unrefined state. Hazelnut oil is mild and easily absorbed so it suits oily or combination skins. It contains useful levels of vitamins and traces of minerals and can be combined with grapeseed or sunflower oil for more economic massage blends.

Johoba oil

This plant oil is in fact a liquid wax and has a superbly light texture. It is similar in text to the skin's own sebum and is one of the best oils to use on the face if your skin-type is combination, oily or prone to acne. Naturally rich in vitamin E, johoba oil has a longer shelf life than many other oils and is an excellent skincare ingredient.

Olive oil

Olive oil is one of the most widely available of all oils and most supermarkets stock cold-pressed (unrefined) versions. Although a fairly sticky oil, olive oil is extremely emollient and useful if your skin is severely dehydrated. Olive oil can be used neat on individual areas of dry skin and is gentle enough to treat children and babies. Naturally enriched with vitamin E and lecithin, olive oil is also an excellent treatment for chapped hands or for soothing sore and inflamed skin.

Passionflower oil

An excellent source of essential fatty acids, vitamin E and traces of minerals, passionflower oil helps to maintain skin elasticity and is useful when applied to the surface of the skin in a massage oil. Most commonly available in capsule form, the contents can be added to enrich many facial oil blends.

Peachnut oil

This plant oil has an unusually light texture and can be used instead of apricot kernel oil when making massage blends. A good source of essential fatty acids, peachnut oil is an excellent addition to face and body oils. Peachnut oil is also traditionally associated with the hair and can be used directly on the scalp as a moisturising treatment.

Sunflower oil

This light-textured oil is especially suited to body massage oil blends, although some may find the faintly earthy smell off-putting. Sunflower oil is one of the cheapest natural moisturisers and can be combined with more expensive ingredients such as borage or evening primrose oil to boost its GLA essential fatty acid content.

Wheatgerm oil

This dark and aromatic oil is extremely sticky when used on its own but makes a wonderful addition to any massage oil blend. The richest natural source of vitamin E, wheatgerm oil can be added to all oil blends to increase their shelf-life and delay rancidity. A few drops of wheatgerm oil can be used neat directly on to scar tissue, such as small burns, where it will greatly speed up the healing process. Wheatgerm oil can also be patted around the eye area as an inexpensive and effective night cream. This plant oil is especially good to use on the skin immediately after being out in the sun as its vitamin E is able to penetrate the skin and help fight the damage caused by UV-induced free radicals.

The Essential Oils

Essential oils are the wonderfully fragrant natural extracts derived from the tiny oil glands in a plant's leaves, roots or flowers. Each essential oil has its own characteristic smell and, according to aromatherapists, its own unique therapeutic properties. Essential oils are excellent additions to many facial massage blends for specific skincare benefits and delicious fragrances.

Choose the essential oils best suited to your skin-type from the chart below, but as these are highly concentrated they must be used sparingly. Do not add more than 10 drops of essential oil to each 2 teaspoons (10 ml) of base oil, and do not use essential oils undiluted on the skin, except when dabbing neat lavender or tea-tree oil on to individual spots or pimples. When buying essential oils, look for the words 'pure essential oil' on the label. These are usually sold in tiny bottles with dropper stoppers for accurate measuring. Oils labelled 'aromatherapy oil' or 'fragrance oil' are often already diluted in almond oil and will not give the same benefits as pure essential oils.

Essential oils for facial massage

name	*origin*	*skin-type*
bergamot	citrus rind	combination/oily skins
camomile	dried flowers	sensitive/children's skins
cedarwood	tree bark	combination/oily skins
cypress	leaves and twigs	oily/problem skins
fennel, sweet	seeds	puffy/swollen skins
frankincense	resin	mature/wrinkled skins
geranium	whole plant	all skins, including sensitive
jasmine	fresh flowers	dry/sensitive skins
lavender	fresh flowers	normal/combination skins
lemon	citrus rind	combination/problem skins
mandarin	citrus rind	normal/combination skins
neroli	orange blossom	combination/oily skins
patchouli	dried leaves	normal/combination skins
petitgrain	leaves and twigs	dry/mature/sensitive skins
rose	fresh petals	dry/mature/sensitive skins

rosemary	flowering tops	combination/oily skins
rosewood	bark	normal/combination skins
sandalwood	bark	sensitive/problem skins
tea-tree	leaves and twigs	combination/oily/problem skins
ylang ylang	fresh petals	normal/combination skins

Energising Exercises

Just as regular exercise soon strengthens and sculpts the body, so facial exercises can successfully be used to work-out the face. Facial work-outs are an effective way of strengthening the underlying muscles that support the skin, and can prevent the skin from slackening and sagging as time goes by. These facial exercises will firm the muscles in the face and, practised regularly, can give results that are as good as a face-lift – but without the physical and financial trauma. Facial exercises not only make the skin firmer and smoother but also improve the way we feel – not only because we become happier with the way our faces look but also because some movements affect moods and emotions. American researcher Paul Ekman has linked the mechanics of facial muscle movement and exercise to the autonomic nervous system which controls our heat rate, breathing and other involuntary activities. Smiling seems to slow the pulse and reduce the physical symptoms of nervous tension and stress. The very exercise of smiling – even if you do not feel like it – also makes us feel physically happier. This is due to the brain remembering that this expression has previously been associated with feeling good and it responds by releasing the appropriate neurotransmitters.

The techniques of facial massage and exercise work well together and can be combined to form a quick and easy part of your daily skincare routine. It is best to begin with the massage routine which acts as a warm-up and prepares the face for a more energetic exercise session. Whether your skin is dry, normal or oily, every face responds quickly to these techniques and you will soon notice a marked improvement in your skin's texture, tone and overall elasticity. Designed to bolster the muscles and ligaments that support the face and control facial expressions, these exercises help to wipe away all signs of tension and prevent the face from becoming fixed with a frown or unflattering scowl lines. The following routine is ideal for all ages and boosts the blood supply to assist teenage problems, such as spots and acne, while providing the additional strength and support needed by the more mature complexions. Once you have learnt the routine you can use it anywhere – at your desk, while washing up, even on a train or when a passenger in the car – provided that you don't mind being stared at!

Wipe away 'crows' feet'

1. Begin by opening your eyes as wide as you can in a startled expression. Feel the skin around the temples pull backwards as you stretch the muscles at the edge of your face. Exercise your eyelids by slowly rolling your eyes, firstly in a clockwise, then in an anti-clockwise, direction. Repeat six times on each side.
2. Work-out the eyes and avoid the eye-strain that can lead to crows' feet by 'palming' at frequent intervals throughout the day. This is especially beneficial for those who work in a fixed position for most of the day or who have to stare at a computer screen for longer periods. It is also a useful technique to use in the evening while watching television for prolonged lengths of time. Begin by placing both palms over your eyes and relaxing your face for one minute in total darkness. Remove your hands and blink your eyes for a few moments before repeating.
3. Next, hold a pencil or similar object at a distance of approximately 6 inches (15 cm) away from the tip of your nose. Look at the top of the pencil, then look up and focus your eyes on a point somewhere in the distance (see diagram on page 105). Repeat 10 times. This exercise works on the muscles around the eyes and will help to keep both the eyes and the surrounding skin healthy and strong.
4. Strengthen the ligaments beneath your forehead and the muscles around the browbones by lifting the eyebrows only with a look of surprise. Repeat ten times, isolating the muscles that work the eyebrows and pulling them up as high as you can before relaxing.

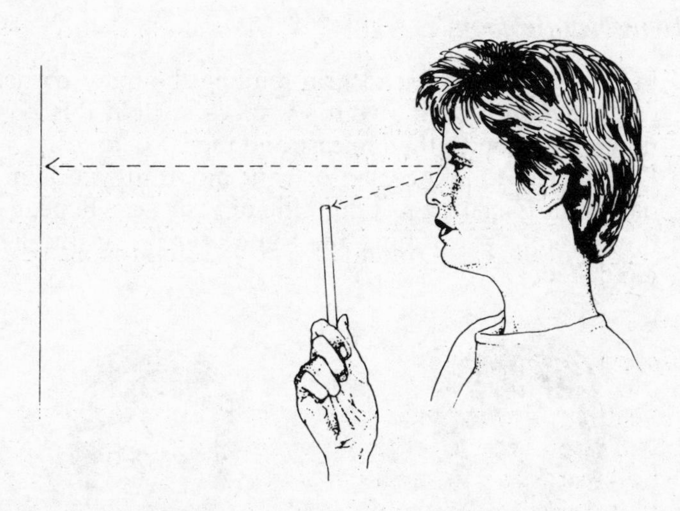

Sculpt the cheekbones

1 Firm the sheet of muscles that cover the cheekbones by lifting the skin that covers the area directly beneath your eyes. Try to isolate the muscles in this part of your face as you pull the skin upwards with a slightly sideways wink. It is worth practising this exercise in the mirror to see the facial muscles working in the correct way before trying on your own. Repeat 10 times on each side.

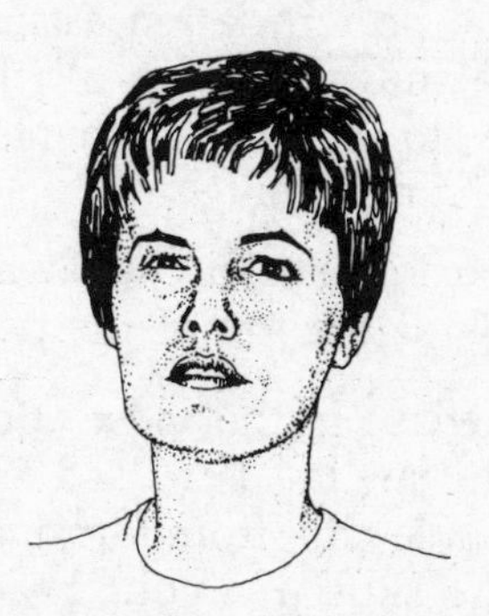

2 Smooth away signs of stress from the sides of the cheeks by twisting the mouth to the left, blocking off the right nostril. Really feel the pull on the right-hand side of your face before relaxing. Repeat ten times before performing the same exercise on the left-hand side of the face.

Strengthen the mouth

1 Begin by giving a broad grin, pulling the outer corners of your mouth back towards your ears. Hold this position for 5 seconds, then release and repeat 10 times.
2 Pull the right-hand corner of your mouth upwards in a half-smile, isolating just one side of your face. Repeat 10 times before performing the same exercise on the left-hand side.

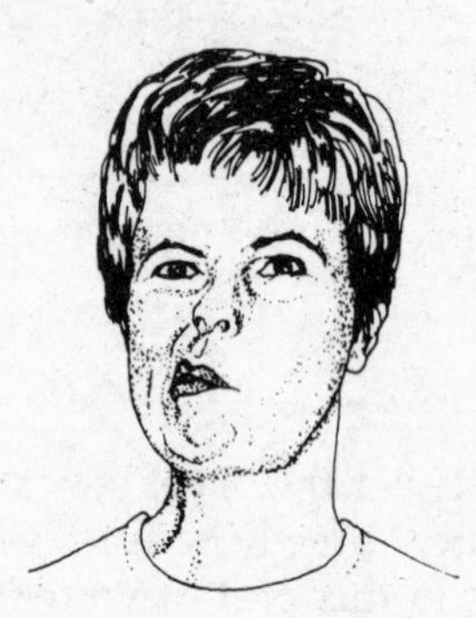

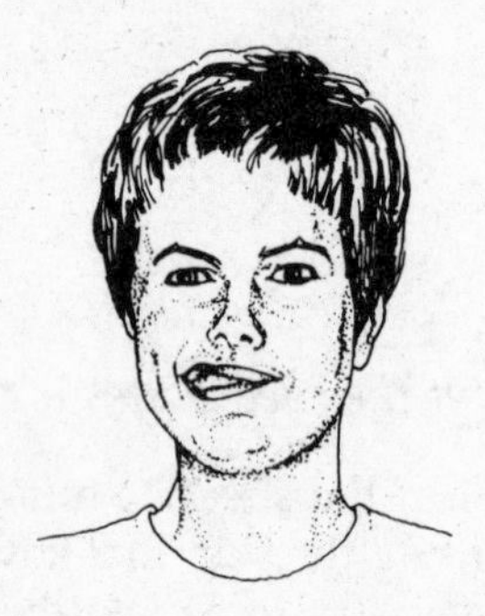

3 Finish the mouth exercises with this one designed to firm the muscles surrounding the lips and jaw area. Silently say the words 'week' and 'queue' alternately, exaggerating the pronunciation as much as possible to achieve the maximum pull on all the muscle groups. Repeat 10 times to feel the ligaments in the upper jaw stretching and strengthening.

Firm a flabby chin

1 This simple exercise is the most effective way to firm and lift a sagging jawline. Practised regularly, it will help to prevent a double-chin from forming and can dramatically tighten the skin. Tip your head backwards until your chin is high in the air. Bring your bottom lip over your top lip and hold it in this 'gurning' position for a count of 5 seconds (see page 95). Repeat at least 10 times, on each occasion pulling the muscles up from the neck and the jaw to encourage the maximum amount of underlying support for the skin.

6

Feed Your Face

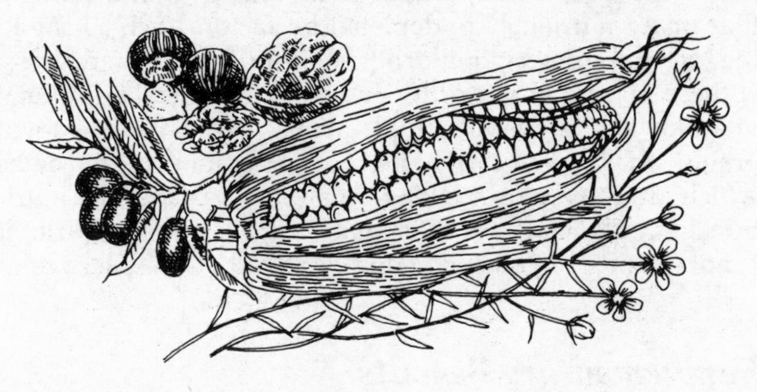

The overall value of a well-balanced diet cannot be over-emphasised in terms of caring for the skin. Just as you cannot run a high-performance car on low-grade fuel without expecting problems, so you cannot expect to have a clear, glowing complexion if you eat junk-food. Instead of foods containing high levels of saturated fat, refined sugar and chemical additives, we need to turn to a diet based on fresh, whole foods prepared with the minimum of processing. It is no coincidence that teenagers, who are notorious for their fast-food eating habits, have some of the worst skins we shall ever see. Unless we lay down the building blocks for better skin from within, our faces will go from pimples to wrinkles in quick succession.

There is one piece of good news here, though, and that is that no matter how badly you have abused your skin from within, it is never too late to change. Because the skin continually sheds dead cells to renew itself every month, it is perfectly possible to improve your complexion dramatically within a few weeks of starting this plan. All you need to do is to add a daily dose of vital oil to your diet, eat far less saturated fat and make sure your foods are fresh and minimally processed to preserve their optimum vitamin and mineral levels.

While the essential fatty acids, vitamin E and lecithin are all important for healthier skin, they cannot function without the presence of many of the other nutrients found in fresh foods. A daily vitamin and mineral supplement can certainly help, but is not the real answer. The best way to better skin is by reassessing your diet and making sure you reach adequate levels of nutrition. Bear in mind, though, that many nutrients are depleted by factors such as smoking, alcohol, prescription drugs, food processing and stress. If these feature in your life, then you may need additional vitamin and mineral supplements. Most better-known brands make well-formulated combinations of nutrients which are often worth taking on a daily basis. While nutritional supplements are safer than drugs, such as aspirin, it is not sensible to exceed the dosage stated on the package.

Supplementary Benefits

Vitamins

Vitamin A (retinol)
Essential for healthy eyesight, skin and for resisting infection, vitamin A keeps the skin elastic and prevents dryness and flakiness. It can help eczema, acne and psoriasis. Deficiency signs include skin disorders and hair loss. Side-effects can occur at daily doses between 10,000–50,000 iu if taken for many months. Retinol comes from animal produce and the best sources are cod liver oil, liver, butter, cheese and eggs.

Vitamin A (beta carotene)
Beta carotene is used by the body to make vitamin A if the body requires additional supplies. It is highly effective at fighting free-radicals and has anti-cancer properties. It is found in all orange-coloured fruit and vegetables and green leafy produce; the best sources are carrots, parsley, spinach, spring greens, sweet potatoes, broccoli and seaweeds.

Vitamin B_1 (thiamin)
This is required to turn carbohydrate into energy and for the nervous system. It can improve mental ability and is destroyed by alcohol. The best sources of vitamin B_1 are yeast, brown rice, wheatgerm, nuts and pork.

Vitamin B_2 (riboflavin)
Vitamin B_2 is essential to convert food into energy and to repair body tissues; it protects the eyes, skin and mucous membranes. Deficiency signs include cracked lips, bloodshot eyes, hair loss, milia (whiteheads) and dizziness. Supplies are depleted by light, heat, smoking and the contraceptive pill. It may harmlessly darken urine or turn it bright yellow. The best sources of vitamin B_2 are yeast, liver, wheatgerm, cheese, eggs, soya flour, yoghurt and leafy vegetables.

Niacin (vitamin B_3)
This vitamin is needed for healthy body tissues and to aid digestion. It also improves the condition of the nails and skin, and can help arthritis and reduce cholesterol. Deficiency signs are insomnia, loss of appetite, dermatitis and skin scaling. High doses of nicotinic acid (above 200 mg daily) can cause skin flushing and depression. Large doses should be avoided during first few months of pregnancy. If taking supplements, look for the safer vitamin form of niacinamide on the label. Best food sources of niacin are yeast, wheat bran, nuts, chicken, oily fish, cheese and dried fruit.

Pantothenic acid (vitamin B_5)
This is important for the nervous system, creating energy, anti-bodies and anti-stress hormones. It is needed for strong, supple skin and can improve dermatitis. Deficiency signs are burning feet and wind pains. Supplies may be depleted by stress, antibiotics, vinegar (pickles, chutneys, etc) and food processing. The best sources are yeast, pig liver, nuts, wheat bran, wheatgerm and eggs.

Vitamin B_6 (pyridoxine)
Essential for the nervous system and healthy skin, vitamin B_6 can also help improve Pre-Menstrual Syndrome, nausea, including morning sickness, and water retention. Deficiency signs are weight gain or a bloated abdomen before periods, dermatitis around the mouth, muscle twitches and irritability. Low levels can lead to dry, oily or scaly skin, dandruff and skin rashes. Supplies may be depleted by oestrogen (the contraceptive pill and hormone replacement therapy), some prescription drugs, alcohol and smoking. The best sources

of vitamin B_6 are brewers' yeast, wheatgerm, oatflakes, bananas, nuts, oily fish, brown rice and vegetables.

Vitamin B_{12} (cyanocobalamin)
This vitamin is needed for energy, DNA and red blood cell production, as well as a healthy nervous system. It can improve brain power and relieve tiredness. Deficiency signs include a sore tongue and menstrual disorders. It may be depleted by alcohol, smoking, antibiotics and alkaline ingredients such as baking powder. Mega-doses are sometimes given by doctors to boost energy. It is most common in animal produce so vegetarians risk a deficiency. The best sources are spirulina algae, pig liver, oily fish, pork, beef, lamb, white fish, eggs, chicken, cheese and alfalfa sprouts.

Folic acid (a B-complex vitamin)
Folic acid is essential for DNA and cell production, and a healthy nervous system. Babies need folic acid to build up a resistance to disease. It can help improve mental health and prevent birth defects (USA recommends taking 800 mcg during pregnancy). It may be depleted by heat (up to 50 per cent lost by boiling vegetables), food processing, alcohol, the contraceptive pill and several other drugs including aspirin. Deficiency signs include greyish-brown pigmentation marks on the skin, hangnails, breathlessness, irritability and confusion. The best sources are yeast, wheatgerm, wheat bran, nuts, pig liver, leafy vegetables, pulses, soya flour and oatflakes.

Biotin (a B-complex vitamin)
Biotin is needed for creating energy, healthy skin, bone marrow and hair, and for regulating the metabolism and hormone production. It can improve skin and scalp problems as well as hair loss, but may be depleted by cooking, antibiotics and stress. Deficiency signs include a pale tongue, skin disorders, including eczema, lethargy, nausea and hair loss. The best sources are yeast, pig liver, eggs, oat flakes, wheat bran, wheatgerm, maize (corn), oily fish and brown rice.

Choline (a B-complex vitamin)
This vitamin is essential for a healthy nervous system, preventing a build-up of blood fats and for healthy cell mainte-

nance. It may be depleted by alcohol. Deficiency signs are raised blood pressure and hardened arteries. It is non-toxic. Best sources are lecithin, liver, egg yolk, steak, wheatgerm, oat flakes, nuts, pulses, citrus fruits and leafy vegetables.

Inositol (a B-complex vitamin)
This vitamin is required to reduce tension, regulate blood fats and maintain healthy hair. It is used as a mild tranquilliser and can improve nerve damage and hair loss. Deficiency signs include eczema, dry skin conditions and falling hair. The best sources are lecithin, liver, wheatgerm, brown rice, oat flakes, steak, citrus fruits, nuts, pulses, bananas and leafy vegetables.

Vitamin C (ascorbic acid)
This anti-oxidant nutrient is essential for the immune system, iron absorption, producing collagen and connective tissue (necessary for soft, smooth skin), regulating cholesterol, producing anti-stress hormones, healthy sexual organs, brain and nerve functions. It can improve colds, influenza, hardened arteries and arthritis, and can reduce levels of toxic metals such as lead and aluminium in the bloodstream. It is depleted by heat, light, air, food processing, the contraceptive pill, aspirin, antibiotics, steroids, stress, smoking and alcohol. Deficiency signs are collagen deterioration resulting in poor skin conditions, premature ageing, general lethargy and haemorrhages, including nosebleeds. Large doses may cause diarrhoea. The best sources are acerola cherries, rosehips, blackcurrants, strawberries, green peppers, broccoli, Brussels sprouts, parsley and citrus fruits.

Bioflavanoids
These are essential for maximising vitamin C and are always found with vitamin C in foods. They are needed to prevent inflammation and infections, and can help menstrual disorders, varicose veins, piles, thrombosis and nosebleeds. They are depleted by the same factors as vitamin C, although they are slightly more stable. Deficiency signs are easy bruising and bleeding. They are non-toxic, and the best sources are citrus fruit skins and pith, lemon juice, apricots, cherries, green peppers, tomatoes and buckwheat.

Vitamin D (calciferol)
Made in the body by processing sunshine through the skin, vitamin D is essential for controlling calcium and phosphate in the body and for healthy bone formation. It is needed to combine with calcium to fight osteoporosis. Deficiency signs are rickets in children and osteomalacia (soft bones) after pregnancy or during old age. It is also thought to be a factor in cancer prevention due to its relationship with calcium absorption. It is especially important that the elderly or housebound obtain vitamin D through their diet as they may not synthesise enough from sunshine. The best sources are sunlight, cod liver oil, and oily fish such as kippers, mackerel, salmon and sardines.

Vitamin E (d-alpha tocopherol)
Vitamin E is essential for the immune system, strong blood capillaries, white blood cells, healthy skin, scar tissue and muscle power. It can help heart disease, skin and menstrual disorders but is depleted by food processing. Deficiency signs include low libido and muscle weakness. The best sources are cold-pressed wheatgerm oil, wheatgerm, unrefined vegetable oils, cod liver oil, peanuts, shrimps, egg yolk, brown rice, salmon, fresh peas and beans.

Vitamin K (phytomenadione)
This vitamin is principally required for blood-clotting and deficiency signs are indicated by haemorrhages (prolonged bleeding) and an inability to form blood clots. Injections of vitamin K are given routinely to new-borns to prevent bleeding from the stomach, intestine and umbilical stump after birth. Babies obtain their own supplies through breast-milk or formula feeds and lactating women are advised to increase their intake to 2–5 mg. Depleted by antibiotics, much remains unknown about this nutrient. The best sources are soyabeans, unrefined vegetable oils, green leafy vegetables, cauliflower and tomatoes.

Minerals

Calcium (Ca)
This is needed for healthy bones, teeth, nerves, muscles and heart functioning. It can help prevent osteoporosis and

allergies. It is depleted by saturated fats, excess dietary fibre, such as bran, and phosphates added to fast food, meat and fizzy drinks. Deficiency signs include bone pain, cramp, 'dowager's hump' and rickets in children. Calcium absorption decreases with age, so the elderly may need to increase their intake to 1,000 mg to maintain balance. Calcium also requires the presence of magnesium in order to function effectively. The best sources of calcium are sesame seeds, seaweeds, almonds, cheese, hazelnuts, parsley, spring greens, soyabeans, yoghurt, milk, fortified brown and white flours.

Magnesium (Mg)
Magnesium is essential for DNA and cell functions, and nerve impulse transmissions. It is needed to metabolise calcium in the body, and can help improve PMT and depression. It is depleted by the contraceptive pill, stress, diuretics, refined and high-sugar foods. Deficiency signs are nervousness, tremors and facial twitches. The best sources are soyabeans, nuts, brewers' yeast, wholemeal flour, seafood and bananas.

Phosphorus (P)
This is required for bone and teeth formation, cellular energy and the nervous system. It improves the absorption of other nutrients from food. Deficiency is rare as junk-foods, including fizzy drinks, are high in phosphates. Meat products may also contain phosphates which are added to soak up additional water. Excess phosphorus leaches calcium from the bones, so post-menopausal women should avoid these foods. The best sources are yeast, dried skimmed milk, wheatgerm, soya flour, cheese, brown rice, wholemeal bread and eggs.

Iron (Fe)
Iron is essential for red blood cell production, a strong immune system and infant development. It is depleted by phytates in raw cereals and wheat bran, phosphates and tannin in tea. Deficiency signs include fatigue, pale inner eyelids and dizziness. Large amount of iron lost during heavy menstrual periods and generally low iron levels

cause anaemia. The USA recommend that the daily intake of iron is increased to 18 mg when breastfeeding. Large amounts can cause constipation. The best sources are yeast, liver, red meat, wheat bran, cocoa, soya flour, parsley, dried fruit, sardines, spinach and wholemeal flour.

Chromium (Cr)
This is required to release energy from glucose, to maintain glucose tolerance, regulate cholesterol and reduce blood fats. It is depleted by sugar and food processing. Deficiency signs include glucose intolerance and high blood fats. Best sources are brewers' yeast, egg yolk, liver, molasses, grapes, mushrooms, asparagus, black pepper, cheese, brown rice, wine, beer, wheatgerm and bran.

Copper (Cu)
This mineral is important for creating melanin (skin pigment) and connective tissues. It improves iron absorption and maintains healthy white blood cells. Deficiency is rare as copper is found in many foods and an excess may do more harm than good. Copper is closely related to zinc and high copper intakes will deplete your levels of zinc. Those with both soft tap water and copper piping will absorb about 1.5 mg daily and should avoid copper in multimineral supplements. The contraceptive pill can increase copper levels and toxicity signs include neausea, stomach and muscle pains and eventually mental disorders. Vitamin C, zinc and manganese reduce copper levels in the body and may be useful supplements to take if your intake is too high. In foods, copper can be found in liver, seafood, brewers' yeast, olives, nuts, lentils, oats and rye. Other, not so welcome, sources include pesticides, copper water pipes and cough medicine.

Manganese (Mn)
Required for a healthy nervous system, thyroid gland and strong bones, manganese levels may be depleted by food processing and excess copper. Deficiencies have been noticed in patients with heart disease and rheumatoid arthritis. Some nutritionists suggest that supplements should be chelated (bound with amino acids) for maximum absorption. The best sources are oats, wheatgerm, whole-

meal bread, avocados, nuts, peas, olives, pineapple, rice, spinach and lettuce.

Molybdenum (Mo)
This is needed to maintain healthy teeth and to regulate iron metabolism. Levels may be depleted by poor or intensively farmed soil. Deficiency signs include an irregular heartbeat and irritability. The best sources are buckwheat, pulses, wheatgerm, liver, barley, lentils, oats, sunflower seeds, offal, wholewheat pasta and eggs.

Selenium (Se)
Selenium is essential for a strong immune system, liver functioning, anti-stress hormones, skin, hair, eyes and heart. It is also effective at removing toxic metals from the body. It may be depleted by poor or intensively farmed soil and acid rain in the soil. Deficiency signs include heart disease, muscle pains, arthritis, cancer, male infertility and hair loss. Areas with high selenium levels in the soil report high birth rates and lower than average cases of cancer and heart disease. Selenium works synergistically with vitamin E and the two nutrients are often found together in supplements for this reason. The best sources of selenium are offal, fish and seafood, meat, whole grains, cereals and dairy produce.

Zinc (Zn)
This is essential for over 200 chemical reactions in the body, including DNA and protein production, insulin and vitamin A mobilisation, healthy glands, sexual development and liver functioning. It is also critical for foetal growth and a child's future learning abilities. It can help acne, eczema, psoriasis, hardening of the arteries, depression, common colds (with vitamin C) and hyperactivity in children. Levels may be depleted by alcohol, the contraceptive pill, smoking, steroids and the phytates in bran. Deficiency signs include white spots on the nails, acne, reduced sense of taste and smell, depression and gynaecological disorders. Some nutritionists suggest that supplements should be chelated (bound with amino acids) for maximum absorption. The best sources are oysters, liver, brewers' yeast, seafood, beef, cheese, sardines, wholemeal bread, eggs, rye bread and chicken.

Food for Thought

A well-balanced diet should include all the nutrients that are so important for creating strong, healthy skin. The recipes on pages 122–145 are to help you get started on the *Save Your Skin* beauty diet. All the recipes are made with fresh, wholesome ingredients that are wonderfully tasty as well as good for the skin. These recipes are also oil-enriched so you will automatically increase your daily intake of essential fatty acids without having to think too hard about it. Most of the recipes rely on minimal cooking or baking at low temperatures to preserve the beneficial qualities of the vegetable oils.

The wholesome ingredients include avocados, nuts and seeds, as these are naturally rich sources of plant oils. However, all saturated fats, including animal produce, have been kept to a minimum. As soon as you start to include the recipes in your daily diet you will notice a distinct improvement in the condition and texture of your skin. The policy for using vital oils in cooking is simple: use at least one tablespoonful of unrefined oil in your foods every day and cut out (or drastically reduce) your intake of saturated fats. You can experiment with your own recipes using many of the different gourmet oils now available, or use these guidelines as a way of increasing your intake of the essential fatty acids.

Weight-watching

Those keeping an eye on their weight and worried about dieting should bear in mind that significant amounts of calories will be saved when cutting down on saturated fats. Oil supplements, such as evening primrose oil and cod liver oil, contain approximately five calories per capsule, so will not ruin even the strictest regime. For cooking, each tablespoonful of vegetable oil contains just 125 calories, which is roughly equivalent to 1 oz (25 g) cheese, ½ pint (300 ml) beer, 4 oz (20 g) salted peanuts or two chocolate digestives, but it is far better for your skin! If you cut all oil out of your diet completely you will not only put your health at risk, but also destroy the basic structure of the skin.

Easy ways to add vital oils

- stir a little hazelnut oil into low-fat hazelnut yoghurt or mix a spoonful into muesli or porridge
- make frothy milk-shakes by liquidising a glass of semi-skimmed milk or soya milk with a dessertspoonful of sunflower oil, adding a banana, low-fat yoghurt and unrefined blackstrap molasses to taste
- use a dessertspoonful of sunflower or safflower oil to glaze vegetables once they have cooked. Simply place the hot vegetables in a bowl, pour on the oil, stir and serve immediately. This is a great way of getting the benefits from the oil without heating them and destroying their chemical structure
- salad dressings are one of the simplest ways to use oils. The basic recipe for a French dressing is two parts olive oil to one part wine vinegar or fresh lemon juice. Season with whole grain mustard, freshly chopped garlic and/or salt and pepper to taste
- dips and sauces are the perfect opportunity for experimenting with delicious gourmet oils. Simply blend a tablespoonful of your favourite vegetable oil (try sesame, walnut or almond for variety) with low-fat soft cheese, cottage cheese, fromage frais or yoghurt. Add seasonings according to taste. Choose tomato purée, whole grain mustard, fresh lemon juice, Tabasco or freshly chopped parsley. Crushed garlic and fresh basil is a delicious combination, or try a dash of soy sauce with freshly grated ginger root for an oriental flavour
- avoid deep-frying as it over-heats the vegetable oil. Many foods can be shallow-fried over a lower heat using olive oil or sesame seed oil. However, even these monounsaturated oils will break down eventually so always throw out any oil that is left in the pan and never reheat it.

Unrefined cooking oils

Although all cooking oils look much the same in the bottle, they are in fact dramatically different – both in taste and health benefits. Another important point to note is that all vegetable oils should be naturally cold-pressed and unrefined. If you can't find either of these words on the bottle, don't buy it! Cold-pressed or unrefined oils contain more of the skin-saving nutrients than processed oils and are far better for the complexion. Cold-pressed oils such as olive oil can be found in most supermarkets now and unrefined oils are commonly available in health food stores. Having made your purchase, store the oil in a cool, dark place such as in the fridge.

These are the vital cooking oils that everybody should get to know:

Corn oil

Corn or maize oil is a good source of polyunsaturated fatty acids and is also one of the cheapest cooking oils available. The oil is extracted from sweetcorn kernels and unfortunately is usually heavily refined before it reaches the shelves (though it is possible to find unrefined versions in health food shops). Unrefined corn oil contains useful levels of vitamin E (66 mg per 100 ml) and, being a polyunsaturated oil, it is a good source of linoleic acid and the other Omega-6 group of essential fatty acids. As with all polyunsaturated oils, corn oil breaks down when heated to high temperatures and produces dangerous free radical peroxides. It is therefore best used cold or warm in recipes such as sauces. Most cooks consider is too heavy to use for salad dressings.

Hazelnut oil

This is a newcomer on the supermarket shelves and has a subtle, nutty flavour. The best hazelnut oil comes from small co-operatives in southern France where it is warm-pressed and filtered by hand. Hazelnut oil is monounsaturated so it can be heated gently without damaging its chemical structure. This light, flavoursome oil can be mixed with a more economical oil, such as sunflower oil, to create delicious salad dressings, or drizzled neat over cheese, baked potatoes or salads.

Olive oil

This is the king of culinary oils and is the most versatile oil of all for cooking. Its fine, light flavour makes it a good base for salad dressings and sauces, and, being monounsaturated, it can also be used for recipes that require heating. It is the only cooking oil I use for frying as it is the most stable vegetable oil when heated to high temperatures. Olive oil is easy to find in its raw, cold-pressed state and most supermarkets sell several different varieties. Avoid the cheaper blends marked 'pure' olive oil as this perversely means that the oil has been refined.

Extra virgin olive oil is taken from the first pressing of olives and has a stronger flavour. It is useful for salad dressings and sauces but too heavy, and too expensive, for everyday frying. Virgin olive oil is a great all-rounder and is taken from the second pressing of the olives. It is lighter in colour and has a milder taste than extra virgin olive oil, but contains just as many essential nutrients. Olive oil is one of the few varieties of oil that can safely be stored in a warm kitchen cupboard as it is one of the most resistant to the effects of rancidity. However, the health-conscious may prefer to keep it in the fridge as the small saturated part of the oil will sink to the bottom of the oil and can be discarded.

Safflower oil

The safflower belongs to the thistle family and was originally cultivated in India where it was also grown for its reddish flowers used to dye cloth vibrant shades of orange and pink. Today, the safflower is grown worldwide for the oil that can be extracted from its crop of tiny seeds. Safflower is one of the most economical cooking oils and can be found in an unrefined state in health food shops. High in polyunsaturates, safflower oil is a good source of linoleic acid and other Omega-6 essential fatty acids, and contains useful levels of vitamin E (49 mg per 100 ml). Safflower oil has a rich, nutty taste and is delicious in salad dressings and sauces. As with other polyunsaturated cooking oils, it should not be used for deep-frying.

Sesame oil

Sesame oil has been used since Roman times as a cooking oil and remains a highly versatile oil that can be used in most recipes. The oil is extracted from the tiny sesame seeds, which are a rich source of calcium and iron. Sesame oil is monounsaturated and so can be more safely heated to high temperatures without the risk of forming toxic elements. A few drops of toasted sesame oil makes a delicious addition to many recipes, but unfortunately the oil has been heavily refined. Unrefined versions of sesame oil are availabe from health food shops. It should always be stored in the fridge.

Sunflower oil

The sunflower is native to Mexico and its botanical name comes from the Greek word for the sun. Sunflowers can grow up to 12 feet (3.6 metres) high and have a large circular seed head surrounded by yellow petals that resemble the sun's rays. Sunflower oil is extracted from the seeds and has a light, slightly sweet taste. The seeds contain about 40 per cent pure oil and are an important crop for farmers in southern France. Sunflower oil is one of the highest in polyunsaturates and the unrefined versions contain useful amounts of linoleic acid and Omega-6 essential fatty acids. Unrefined sunflower oil also contains reasonable amounts of vitamin E (27 mg per 100 ml). Sunflower oil is best used cold in dressings or sauces and, because it contains such high amounts of polyunsaturates, it should definitely be stored in the fridge. I use sunflower oil to make my own healthy spread by blending 1 part oil to 2 parts butter in the food processor. This keeps for several weeks in an airtight container in the fridge (if the oil separates out, simply stir it back in).

Walnut oil

Walnut oil is another French newcomer to our supermarket shelves and may also be labelled as *Huile de Noix*, or *Huile de Noix Extra* (a slightly stronger flavour). Traditionally, French chefs use it for frying delicacies and it gives a delicious flavour to fried eggs, omelettes and wild mushrooms. Unrefined walnut oil is easy to find as most is produced by the traditional cold-pressed method and simply filtered before being bottled. Although more expensive than other cooking oils, a few drops go a long, long way and are a tasty addition to many recipes. Unopened walnut oil will keep for up to a year (check the bottle for a bottling date) and once open should be stored in the fridge.

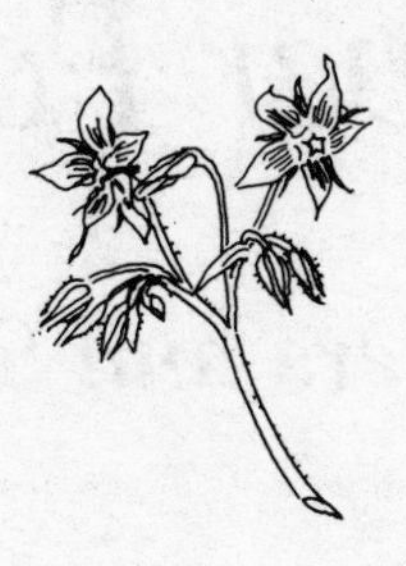

Skin Saving Super Foods

Starters and Snacks

Chilled Cucumber Soup

A refreshing summer starter, the flavour of this soup develops if it is made the day before it is required.

Serves 4–6

1 small onion, finely chopped
1 garlic clove, crushed
2 large cucumbers, peeled and finely chopped
3 tablespoons olive or sesame oil
1 tablespoon chopped fresh tarragon or 1 teaspoon dried tarragon
1 tablespoon tarragon or cider vinegar
5 tablespoons dry white wine
½ pint (300 ml) chicken or vegetable stock
4 tablespoons low-fat fromage frais
salt and pepper
slivers of lemon peel and cucumber skin, to garnish

Sauté the onion, garlic and cucumber in the olive or sesame oil for about 5 minutes or until soft. Add the tarragon and season with salt and pepper. Pour in the vinegar and white wine, bring to the boil, then reduce the heat, cover and simmer over a low heat for about 20 minutes. Purée the mixture in a blender or food processor, or pass it through a fine sieve. Stir in the chicken or vegetable stock and refrigerate for 2–3 hours or until completely chilled. Just before serving, stir in the fromage frais. Serve garnished with slivers of lemon peel and cucumber skin.

Gazpacho

Serves 4

6 large tomatoes, finely chopped
½ onion, finely diced
1 green pepper, de-seeded and finely chopped
½ cucumber, diced
2 garlic cloves, chopped
4 tablespoons unrefined sunflower oil
2 tablespoons hazelnut or walnut oil
3 tablespoons wine vinegar or blackcurrant vinegar
½ pint (300 ml) chilled chicken or vegetable stock
salt and pepper
For the garnish:
4 teaspoons low-fat yoghurt or fromage frais
1 tablespoon finely chopped chives

Put the chopped vegetables, garlic and herbs in a non-metallic dish and pour in the sunflower and nut oils, and vinegar. Leave to marinate in the fridge for at least 30 minutes (the longer you can leave the flavours to steep, the better it will taste). Remove the vegetables from the fridge, pour over the stock, season with salt and pepper, and stir well. Serve chilled, garnished with a spoonful of low-fat yoghurt or fromage frais and a sprinkling of chopped chives.

Avocado Soup

Serves 6

2 medium onions, chopped
2 garlic cloves, chopped
2 tablespoons olive oil
2 pints (1.2 litres) chicken or vegetable stock
2 medium avocados
grated rind and juice of 1 lime
salt and pepper
Greek yoghurt or low-fat fromage frais, to garnish

Fry the onion and garlic in the olive oil for about 5 minutes or until translucent. Add the chicken or vegetable stock, season with salt and pepper and bring to the boil. Reduce the heat, cover and simmer for 30 minutes. Meawhile, halve, stone and peel the avocados.

Mash or purée the avocados with the lime juice and rind and stir this into the soup. Warm through and serve with a spoonful of Greek yoghurt or low-fat fromage frais stirred into each bowl.

Avocado Dip

Serves 2–3 as a starter

1 large ripe avocado
2 tablespoons lime or lemon juice
2 tablespoons olive oil
¼ teaspoon chopped fresh or dried oregano
salt and peper
To serve:
carrots, radishes and celery, prepared as necessary

Halve, stone and peel the avocado and mash the flesh with a fork, or purée it in a blender, with the lime or lemon juice. Gradually stir in the oil, and blend until smooth. Add the oregano and season with pepper and the minimum of salt.

Cut the carrots and celery into matchsticks and halve or quarter the radishes if they are large. Put the dip in a bowl, stand it in the centre of a large plate and surround it with the vegetable crudités. Serve as a light starter or party snack.

Olive Oil Bread

This traditional Provençale recipe makes a rich, heavy bread perfect for serving with soups or vegetable pâtés, or spread with sun-dried tomato paste. Making this bread could be considered a beauty treatment in itself, as the kneading action is terrific exericse for the hands and the olive oil leaves them feeling amazingly soft.

Makes 2 large loaves

½ oz (15 g) fresh yeast or 1½ teaspoons dried yeast
½ teaspoon sugar
½ pint (300 ml) warm water
1 lb (450 g) strong wholemeal bread flour (preferably organically grown), or 8 oz (225 g) strong wholemeal bread flour and 8 oz (225 g) strong white bread flour
8 tablespoons olive oil
¼ teaspoon ascorbic acid (vitamin C) powder
1 tablespoon chopped fresh oregano or ½ teaspoon freeze-dried oregano
1 tablespoon chopped fresh basil or ½ tablespoon freeze-dried basil
2 tablespoons chopped black olives (optional)
2 tablespoons chopped onion (optional)

Mix the fresh yeast with the sugar and a small amount of the warm water and leave to stand for 10 minutes or until frothy. Alternatively, prepare the dried yeast according to packet instructions.

Sift the flours into a large bowl, adding the bran left in the sieve after sifting the wholemeal flour. Pour in the yeast mixture and add the remaining water, 1 tablespoon of the olive oil and the ascorbic acid (vitamin C) powder. Knead well until the dough is smooth and elastic. Alternatively, combine the ingredients in a food processor using a dough hook or plastic blade. Place the dough in an oiled bowl, cover with a clean cloth and leave in a warm place to rise for at least 20 minutes or until doubled in size.

Knead the dough again by hand, adding the herbs and the remaining olive oil. Work the oil well into the dough to distribute it evenly thoughout the bread. Add the chopped black olives and/or onion, if using. Divide the dough into two roughly equal portions and mould into flat circular shapes. Using a sharp knife, score a cross on the top of each loaf to make the bread easier to break into portions once cooked. Place on a greased baking tray, cover with a clean cloth and leave to rise for a second time. Bake in the oven at 220°C/425°F/gas mark 7 for approximately 20 minutes or until crisp and brown. Serve warm.

Family Fare

Pumpkin Pilaff with Pumpkin Seeds

Serves 2

6 oz (175 g) long-grain rice (or a mixture of long-grain and wild rice)
4 tablespoons olive oil
1 onion, chopped
6–8 no-soak dried apricots, thinly sliced
1 lb (450 g) peeled pumpkin, de-seeded
1 green pepper, de-seeded
2 oz (50 g) soft brown sugar
4 oz (100 g) pumpkin seeds

Heat 1 tablespoon of the oil in a deep saucepan, add the onion and fry for 5 minutes or until translucent. Rinse the rice thoroughly and add to the onion. Stir until all the rice is coated with oil, then add twice the volume of water as there is rice. Bring to the boil, then reduce the heat and simmer for 10 minutes. Add the apricots and cook for a further 5 minutes.

Drain the rice and rinse under cold running water. Slice the pumpkin and the green pepper into bite-sized chunks. Add half the pumpkin and all the pepper to the rice mixture, together with half the sugar, 1 tablespoon of the remaining olive oil and the pumpkin seeds. Place in a greased ovenproof dish and arrange the remaining pumpkin over the top. Brush with the remaining oil and sprinkle over the rest of the sugar. Cover and bake in a preheated oven at 180°C/350°F/gas mark 4 for 40–45 minutes.

Baked Fish with Pine Nut and Garlic Sauce

Serves 6

1½ –2 lb (700–900 g) fillets of fish, such as mackerel, herring, trout or cod
juice of ½ lemon
1 tablespoon olive oil

chopped fresh parsley
salt and pepper

For the sauce:
4 oz (100 g) pine nuts
2 garlic cloves, crushed
2 tablespoons lemon juice
2 tablespoons olive oil
salt and pepper

Place the fish fillets in an ovenproof dish, sprinkle over the lemon juice, olive oil and parsley, and season with salt and pepper. Cover and bake in the oven at 180°C/350°F/gas mark 5 for 20–30 minutes or until the fish is cooked through.

Meanwhile, place the pine nuts and garlic in a food processor or blender, season with salt and pepper and process until fairly smooth. Slowly trickle in the lemon juice, then the olive oil, and continue to process until the sauce is thick and creamy. Pour the sauce over the fish and return to the oven to heat through, or reheat in a saucepan and serve as a separate accompaniment.

Mighty Mince

This recipe feeds a hungry family and replaces the saturated animal fat normally found in minced meat with much healthier vegetable oils. Serve with baked potatoes or pasta shells and peas.

Serves 3–4

8 oz (225 g) lean minced beef or lamb
3 tablespoons olive, unrefined sunflower or safflower oil
4 leeks, thinly slices
4 medium carrots, thinly sliced
pinch each of dried rosemary and oregano
14 oz (400 g) can chopped tomatoes
salt and pepper

Cook the mince in a microwave oven or in a saucepan on the hob for about 10 minutes or until browned. Drain off all the meat juices and fat and discard.

Gently heat the oil over a low heat, add the leeks and carrots, and simmer for 5 minutes or until the vegetables are just soft. Add the drained mince and all the remaining ingredients, and bring to the boil, then reduce the heat, cover and simmer over a low heat for a further 5–10 minutes to allow the flavours to develop.

Cheesy Herbed Pasta

Serves 4–6

4 tablespoons olive or sesame oil
6 beef or extra large tomatoes, skinned and sliced
2 garlic cloves, crushed
2 courgettes, diced
14 oz (400 g) fresh pasta shapes (shells, spirals or quills, etc)
6 oz (175 g) buffalo mozzarella (made with buffalo milk) or 6 oz (175 g) ricotta cheese
a handful of fresh basil leaves
freshly ground black pepper
2 oz (50 g) freshly grated Parmesan cheese, to serve (optional)

Gently heat the oil in a large saucepan and add the tomatoes and garlic. Add the courgettes and simmer for 10 minutes or until the vegetables are soft.

Meanwhile, cook the pasta in a large saucepan of rapidly boiling water, with a dash of olive oil added, for 4–6 minutes or until *al dente* (tender but still slightly firm to the bite). Take care not to overcook.

Drain the pasta and stir it into the vegetables, adding the chopped mozzarella or ricotta cheese, the basil leaves and black pepper just before serving. Serve with a sprinkling of freshly grated Parmesan, if liked.

Aubergine, Mushroom and Hazelnut Pâté

Serve this tasty pâté surrounded by a green salad together with toasted fingers of warm pitta bread as a starter, or as the main dish for a light lunch.

Serves 2 as a main course; 4 as a starter

1 medium aubergine
3 tablespoons hazelnut oil
2 oz (50 g) unsalted butter
4 oz (100 g) mushrooms, chopped
2 garlic cloves
2 oz (50 g) hazelnuts
2 teaspoons tomato purée
1 teaspoon chopped fresh thyme
juice of ½ lemon
salt and pepper

Split the aubergine in half lengthways and brush the white flesh with 1 tablespoon of the oil. Bake in the oven at 180°C/350°F/gas mark 4 for 20 minutes or until the flesh is soft.

Melt the butter in a saucepan, add the mushrooms and garlic, and fry lightly until they are quite soft. Scoop the flesh out of the aubergine halves and cut it into small cubes. Put the hazelnuts in a food processor and process until fairly finely chopped. Add the mushrooms, tomato purée, thyme, lemon juice and aubergine flesh. Season with salt and pepper, then blend well until smooth, spoon into individual ramekin dishes and refrigerate.

Stuffings, Sauces and Dressings

Ginger and Apricot Stuffing

This stuffing is a delicious filling for fresh poultry and game, or can be shaped into small patties and shallow-fried in olive oil to serve as an accompaniment to lean lamb or pork chops.

Makes enough to stuff one chicken or to serve 6 as a condiment

1 slice of wholemeal bread, crusts removed
2 oz (50 g) no-soak dried apricots, chopped
1 oz (25 g) fresh parsley or coriander, chopped

2 oz (50 g) mushrooms, finely sliced
1 oz (25 g) fresh ginger root, chopped or grated
4 tablespoons olive or sesame oil

Chop or grate the bread into fine breadcrumbs, or whizz in a blender until turned to crumbs. Add all the remaining ingredients and mix well.

Almond and Tomato Mayonnaise

Serve this mayonnaise with salad leaves or drizzle over baked potatoes and pasta.

Serves 2–4

2 oz (50 g) ground almonds
4 oz (100 g) fresh tomatoes, skinned
1 garlic clove
1 egg
1 teaspoon French mustard
1 teaspoon white wine vinegar
7 fl oz (200 ml) unrefined oil (try a mixture of corn and nut oil)
salt and pepper

Place all the ingredients, except the oil, in a food processor and process until fairly smooth. With the processor still running, trickle the oil gradually through the funnel and continue to whizz until the mayonnaise has become thick and creamy.

Deliciously Mild Curry Sauce

Serve this sauce with stir-fried vegetables and rice or couscous, or add chunks of fish, chicken or tofu to make a spicy casserole.

Serves 2–4

4 oz (100 g) finely chopped onion
4 tablespoons sunflower or sesame oil

2 teaspoons mild curry powder
1 teaspoon honey
2 tablespoons freshly ground hazelnuts, peanuts or pecans, or 2 tablespoons peanut or hazelnut butter
2 garlic cloves, crushed
pinch of sea salt
grated rind and juice of ½ lemon
¾ pint (450 ml) leftover vegetable water or stock
freshly ground black pepper

Gently sauté the chopped onion in the oil over a low heat. Stir in the curry powder and heat through. Add the honey, nuts or nut butter, garlic, salt, lemon juice and lemon rind. Reduce the heat, stir in the vegetable water or stock and season with black pepper.

Peanut Satay Sauce

This wonderfully simple sauce transforms skewers of chicken, fish or lean lamb into exotic sticks of satay. Serve accompanied by slices of fresh cucumber and spring onions.

Serves 2–4

6 oz (175 g) unsalted peanuts (preferably freshly shelled)
½ teaspoon sea salt
1 teaspoon unrefined sesame oil
3 tablespoons unrefined sunflower or safflower oil
1 small onion, finely chopped
4 tablespoons lemon juice
3 garlic cloves, crushed
1 dried red chilli, de-seeded and crushed (optional)
6–8 tablespoons water

Place all the ingredients, except the water, in a food processor and whizz until smooth. Thin the sauce by adding a few drops of water until the desired consistency is achieved. Allow to stand for at least 1 hour for the flavours to develop before using. Serve in individual bowls alongside grilled fish or meat skewers.

Light Lunches and Side Dishes

Cracked Wheat with Herbs

Serve as an accompaniment to meat or fish in place of potatoes.

Serves 4

8 oz (225 g) cracked wheat
3 tablespoons olive or sesame oil
2 onions, finely chopped
1 garlic clove, crushed (optional)
1 tablespoon chopped fresh basil or parsley
2½ pints (1.4 litres) boiling water

In a large saucepan, sauté the cracked wheat in the olive or sesame oil until it begins to brown. Add the onions, garlic, if using, and herbs. Stir in the boiling water, cover and simmer for 5 minutes or until all the water has been absorbed and the wheat is soft and fluffy, stirring occasionally.

Mushrooms Stuffed with Cheese and Nuts

A winner with vegetarians, this dish may be served hot as a side-dish to a sit-down dinner, or as one of the dishes for an informal buffet.

Serves 4

8 oz (225 g) medium mushrooms, wiped
1 small onion
2 garlic cloves
1 tablespoon walnut, hazelnut or almond oil
3 oz (75 g) freshly chopped hazelnuts and almonds
2 oz (50 g) fresh breadcrumbs
2 oz (50 g) half-fat Cheddar cheese

Remove the mushroom stalks and chop them finely with the onion. Crush the garlic over the mixture and mix well.

Heat the nut oil in a saucepan and fry the chopped mixture for a few minutes or until the onion becomes transparent. Remove from the heat and stir in the chopped nuts, breadcrumbs and cheese. Use the mixture to stuff (but not overfill) the mushroom cups. Place on an oiled baking tray and cook in the oven at 190°C/375°F/gas mark 5 for 20 minutes.

Tabouleh Parcels

This traditional savoury dish is pretty enough to present at a smart dinner party and is delicious served hot with vegetables or cold with a salad.

Serves 6

8 oz (225 g) fine bulgar wheat
1 large onion, finely chopped
1 oz (25 g) chopped fresh parsley
4 tablespoons chopped fresh mint
4 tablespoons unrefined sunflower or safflower oil
4 tablespoons lemon juice
12 large lettuce leaves
6 long fresh chives
salt and pepper

Soak the wheat and chopped onion for at least 1 hour, or even overnight, in hot water, then press the plumped-up grains in a sieve to remove excess moisture. Stir in the chopped herbs, oil and lemon juice, and season with salt and pepper.

Blanch the lettuce leaves briefly in boiling water, then drain and cool. When cool, spread each leaf out flat on a chopping board and place a spoonful of tabouleh mixture on to each one. Fold the lettuce leaf over the mixture to form a fat parcel and tie with a fresh chive.

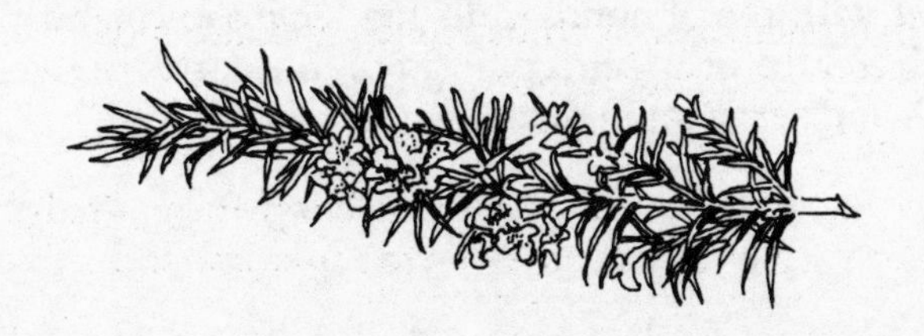

Gingered Carrots

This recipe is a really delicious way of serving an ordinary root vegetable. The method works as well for yams and parsnips.

Serves 4

1½ lb (700 g) carrots, diced
2 tablespoons sesame or hazelnut oil
¼ teaspoon grated fresh root ginger
½ teaspoon arrowroot or kuzu, mixed with 3 tablespoons water
5 tablespoons water or vegetable stock
salt and pepper
chopped fresh parsley, to garnish

Sauté the carrot in the oil. Add the water or stock and grated ginger, cover and simmer until tender. Stir in the diluted arrowroot or kuzu and simmer for another 1–2 minutes or until smooth and creamy. Season with salt and pepper, sprinkle with chopped parsley and serve immediately.

Steamed Broccoli with Olive Oil, Lemon and Almonds

Serves 4

1 lb (450 g) broccoli
2 tablespoons olive oil
2 oz (50 g) slivered almonds
juice of ½ lemon

Separate the broccoli into florets and steam for 5–8 minutes or until bright green and just tender. Meanwhile, mix the olive oil with the almonds, add the lemon juice and warm through gently in a saucepan. Pour the mixture over the broccoli and serve immediately.

New Potatoes with Avocado Sauce

This smooth and creamy avocado sauce can also be served with many types of vegetables, plain grilled chicken or fish.

Serves 4–6

1½–2 lb (700–900 g) new potatoes
1 medium onion
2 tablespoons olive oil
2 medium ripe avocados
juice of 1 lime
5 sprigs of fresh coriander
2 tablespoons low-fat fromage frais
sea salt and pepper

Steam the new potatoes or cook in boiling salted water until tender. Meanwhile, fry the onion in the olive oil for about 5 minutes or until translucent. Place in a food processor. Halve, peel and stone the avodacos and roughly chop the flesh. Add to the onion with the lime juice and coriandor stems and leaves (reserving a few of the leaves for garnish). Season with sea salt and pepper and blend all the ingredients until smooth.

Empty the sauce back into the saucepan, warm through and stir in the fromage frais. Serve poured over the warm potatoes and garnish with the reserved coriander.

Cauliflower Curry with Cashews

Serves 4

1 tablespoon sesame oil
1 large onion, chopped
2 garlic cloves, chopped
½ teaspoon ground turmeric
½ teaspoon ground cumin
1 teaspoon ground coriander seeds
1 fresh green chilli, de-seeded and chopped
4 oz (100 g) cashew nuts
1 cauliflower, divided into florets

Heat the oil gently in a saucepan and fry the garlic and onion for about 5 minutes or until translucent. Stir in the turmeric, cumin, coriander, chilli and cashews and cook for a further 1 minute, then add the cauliflower and 4 tablespoons water. Cover and simmer for 20 minutes, checking during cooking that the liquid does not boil away completely. Serve immediately.

Chicken and Almond Fingers

The chicken can be minced in a food processor fitted with a metal chopping blade.

Serves 4–6

4 tablespoons olive oil
1 lb (450 g) filo pastry, thawed if frozen
For the filling:
8 oz (225 g) minced chicken
4 oz (100 g) chopped almonds
2 tablespoons lemon juice
1 garlic clove, crushed
1 teaspoon paprika
¼ teaspoon ground cumin

Prepare the filling simply by incorporating all the ingredients in a bowl and stirring thoroughly. Divide each sheet of filo pastry into two rectangles. Make sure that the pastry not in immediate use is kept covered, preferably with a damp cloth, as it dries out very quickly.

Starting with one of the rectangles of pastry, brush the whole sheet with the olive oil. Place 1–2 teaspoons of the chicken mixture along the centre of the short edge. Fold in the two long sides to cover the chicken mixture and roll up like a cigar. Continue in this way until all the chicken mixture has been used. Place the chicken 'fingers' on a greased baking tray, with the edges folded underneath to help seal them. Brush with the remaining oil and bake in the oven at 190°C/375°F/gas mark 5 for 20–25 minutes or until the pastry is golden and the chicken is cooked through. Serve hot.

Superb Salads

Caesar Salad with Nuts and Nut Oil Dressing

This dish needs no additional salt because of the saltiness of the anchovies, even though much of this is removed by soaking them in milk.

Serves 4

1 Cos lettuce
3 oz (75 g) hazelnuts or walnut, chopped
3 oz (75 g) freshly grated Parmesan cheese
For the dressing:
1 egg, size 2
3 tablespoons walnut or hazelnut oil
4 anchovies, soaked in milk to remove excess salt, drained and finely chopped
4 capers, chopped
1 garlic clove, crushed
freshly ground black pepper

To make the dressing, place the walnut or hazelnut oil in a screw-topped jar with the garlic, anchovy fillets, capers and some freshly ground black paper. Par-boil the egg for 1 minute and break this into the jar. Shake together very thoroughly to form a smooth, rich dressing. Alternatively, place all the dressing ingredients in a food processor fitted with a metal chopping blade and process until smooth.

Tear the lettuce leaves into bite-sized pieces and put them in a serving bowl. Pour over the dressing, sprinkle the nuts and cheese over, and toss together with the dressing. Serve immediately.

Date, Apple and Hazelnut Salad

To prevent the pieces of chopped apple turning brown, have ready a bowl of water to which some lemon juice has been added. Drop the apple into this as you cut them up.

Serves 4–6

1 lb (450 g) crisp eating apples, cored and chopped
8 oz (225 g) dates (preferably fresh), stoned and halved
4 oz (100 g) hazelnuts

For the dressing:
5 fl oz (140 ml) carton low-fat natural yoghurt
1 tablespoon sunflower oil
1 teaspoon honey
1 teaspoon mustard
salt and pepper

Just before serving, drain the apple pieces and mix them with the dates and hazelnuts. To make the dressing, mix all the ingredients together. Stir spoonfuls of the dressing into the salad according to taste.

Avocado, Tomato, Baked Pepper and Spring Onion Salad

Serves 4

1 yellow pepper
1 red or green pepper
1 large avocado
8 oz (225 g) firm ripe tomatoes, thinly sliced
3 spring onions, sliced

For the dressing:
3 tablespoons olive oil
1 tablespoon white wine vinegar
1 tablespoon honey
1 teaspoon mustard
1 tablespoon chopped fresh basil (optional)
salt and pepper

Put the peppers in an ovenproof dish with about 1 inch (2.5 cm) cold water in the bottom. Bake in the oven at 190°C/375°F/gas mark 5 for about 40 minutes or until soft, turning the peppers several times during cooking. (This can also be done much more quickly in a microwave.) Drain the water from the dish, cover the peppers with a lid or cloth and leave to cool. When cold, peel and de-seed the peppers and cut into thin strips.

Halve, stone and peel the avocado and slice the flesh thinly. Arrange the avocado and tomato slices alternately overlapping each other on a flat dish. Arrange the peppers around the edge of the dish and sprinkle the spring onions over the other vegetables. Combine the dressing ingredients, pour over the salad and serve.

Hot Bean Salad with Peanuts

Serves 6

1 lb (450 g) green beans (haricot, Kenya, etc)
15 oz (430 g) can red kidney beans, drained and rinsed
4 oz (100 g) unsalted peanuts
2 spring onions, finely sliced, to garnish

For the dressing:
3 tablespoons peanut (ground nut) oil
1 tablespoon lemon juice
1 garlic clove, crushed
salt and pepper

Top and tail the green beans and place in a pan of boiling water. Cook for 10 minutes or until just tender. Put the dressing ingredients in a screw-topped jar, close firmly and shake until all the ingredients are combined. Drain the beans and mix with the kidney beans and nuts. Pour the dressing over, toss well and garnish with the onion rings.

Gourmet Chick-pea and Tuna Salad

This dish is based on a Greek dish called *skepastaria,* from the island of Sifnos, where the women take their casseroles of chick-peas to the communal village oven for baking. It tastes best if you have the time to prepare the dried chick-peas one day in advance; otherwise two 14 oz (400 g) cans of chick-peas may be used instead. Serve with a green salad.

Serves 4–6

14 oz (400 g) dried chick-peas, soaked overnight in cold water, or 2 × 14 oz (400 g) can chick-peas, drained and rinsed
5 tablespoons olive oil
1 onion, roughly chopped
1 bay leaf
2 garlic cloves

For the tuna:
3 tablespoons olive oil
8 oz (225 g) fresh tuna, cut into chunks, or 8 oz (225 g) can tuna, packed in brine
2 tablespooons dry sherry or Japanese mirin flavouring

For the salad dressing:
6 tablespoons olive oil
2 tablespoons lemon juice
2 large tomatoes, skinned and chopped
3 small red onions, finely diced
2 oz (50 g) pitted black olives
2 oz (50 g) pitted green olives
salt and pepper

Drain the dried chick-peas, put them in a large saucepan, cover with fresh water and bring to the boil. Boil rapidly for 15 minutes, then transfer the chick-peas to a deep casserole and add the olive oil, onion, bay leaf and whole, skinned garlic cloves. Add enough water to cover the chick-peas by about ½ inch (1 cm) and bake in the oven at 120°C/250°F/gas mark 1–2 for at least 6 hours or overnight. In the morning, remove the chopped onion, bay leaf and garlic and the chick-peas are ready to use.

To make the salad dressing, mix the olive oil with the lemon juice, tomatoes and stir in the olives and season.

To cook the tuna, heat the olive oil in a frying pan or wok, add the tuna and fry until lightly browned. Add the sherry or mirin and cook for a further 2–3 minutes. Combine the cooked tuna with the chick-peas and pour over the salad dressing. Mix well and serve warm.

Puddings and Cakes

Sesame Seed Cookies

As an occasional treat, these crumbly cookies are far better for you than those made with animal fats or hydrogenated oils. A favourite with children of all ages, these biscuits are also dairy-free.

Makes about 36 cookies

4 heaped tablespoons honey
4 heaped tablespoons unrefined blackstrap molasses
¼ pint (150 ml) sesame or hazelnut oil
pinch of sea salt
8 oz (225 g) sesame seeds
4 oz (100 g) rolled oats
4 oz (100 g) soya flour
3 oz (75 g) wholemeal flour
1 tablespoon grated orange rind
1 tablespoon fresh orange juice

Cream together the honey, molasses, oil and salt. Stir in the sesame seeds, oats, flours, grated orange rind and orange juice. Mix well and spread in a well-oiled 9 × 12 inch (22 × 30 cm) baking tin. Bake in the oven at 180°C/350°F/gas mark 3 for 15 minutes or until golden brown. Cut into squares and leave to cool. Store in an airtight container.

Honey and Almond Biscuits

Makes about 24 biscuits

2 oz (50 g) butter
1 tablespoon olive oil
2 tablespoons vanilla caster sugar
1 tablespoon honey

2 oz (50 g) ground almonds
4 oz (100 g) plain flour
4 oz (100 g) chopped almonds

Put the butter, olive oil and sugar in a food processor and process until light and fluffy. Add the honey, ground almonds and flour and process until well blended. Stir in the chopped almonds. Roll the mixture into small balls and place, well spaced apart, on an oiled baking sheet. Flatten each ball slightly, then bake in the oven at 150°C/300°F/gas mark 2 for 35–40 minutes. Cool on a wire rack and store in an airtight container.

Low-fat Strawberry and Nut Cheesecake

Lower in animal fat and higher in plant oils than most recipes, this cheesecake is a delicious special occasion pudding.

Serves 6–8

For the base:
3 oz (75 g) wholemeal digestive biscuits, broken into pieces
1½ oz (40 g) hazelnuts
1½ oz (40 g) almonds
3 tablespoons almond or hazelnut oil
1 oz (25 g) butter
2 oz (50 g) brown sugar
For the cheese mixture:
10 fl oz (280 ml) low-fat fromage frais
6 oz (175 g) half-fat cream cheese
6 oz (175 g) low-fat quark or curd cheese
grated rind and juice of 1 lemon
2 eggs, size 3, separated
½ oz (15 g) powdered gelatine
For the topping:
4–6 oz (100–175 g) strawberries
2 oz (50 g) slivered almonds

To make the base, put the broken biscuits, hazelnuts and almonds in a food processor and process for 20 seconds.

Gently heat the oil, butter and sugar in a saucepan until the butter has melted and the sugar has dissolved. Pour this into the food processor and process for a further 5–10 seconds until it has completely combined. Spread the mixture in the base of an 8 inch (20.5 cm) loose-bottomed cake tin and chill until firm.

Meanwhile, place the fromage frais, cream cheese, quark (or curd cheese), lemon juice and rind and egg yolks in the processor. Put the gelatine in a saucepan with 3 tablespoons water and heat gently until the gelatine dissolves. Pour this into the processor with the other ingredients and process for 30 seconds. Whisk the egg whites until stiff and fold them into the cheese mixture. Pour over the biscuit base and refrigerate until set. Decorate the finished cheesecake with slivered almonds and strawberries.

Flapjacks with Nuts and Ginger

Makes about 20 flapjacks

4 oz (100 g) butter
3 oz (75 g) soft brown sugar
1 tablespoon honey
1 tablespoon hazelnut oil (plus a little extra for greasing the tin)
6 oz (175 g) rolled oats
4 oz (100 g) chopped mixed nuts
½ teaspoon ground ginger
¼ teaspoon salt

Grease a tin measuring about 8" × 10" (16 × 26 cm) with a little of the oil. Beat the butter, sugar, honey and nut oil together until the mixture is creamy. Mix together the rolled oats, nuts, ginger and salt and work into the sugar and butter mixture. Put this mixture into the tin and press down well. Bake in the oven at 180°C/350°F/gas mark 4 for 30–40 minutes.

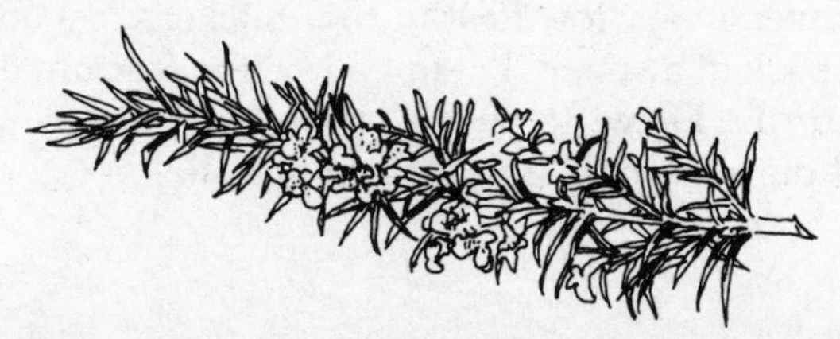

Carrot Cake

Makes one 7 inch (15 cm) cake

2 eggs, size 3
6 oz (175 g) brown sugar
¼ pint (150 ml) walnut or hazelnut oil
2 tablespoons honey
2 oz (50 g) chopped walnuts
8 oz (225 g) plain flour
8 oz (225 g) finely grated carrots
4 tablespoons orange juice
grated rind of 2 oranges
1 teaspoon bicarbonate of soda

Whisk the eggs and sugar together until pale and fluffy, then gradually whisk in the oil. Fold in all the other ingredients and pour into an oiled and lined 7 inch (15 cm) cake tin. Bake in the oven at 180°C/350°F/gas mark 4 for 50 minutes–1 hour or until a skewer inserted in the centre comes out clean. Leave to cool in the tin for 10 minutes before tipping out on to a wire cake rack to cool completely.

Low-fat Chestnut Ice-Cream

Serves 4

½ pint (300 ml) skimmed milk
3 eggs, size 3, separated
3 oz (75 g) caster sugar
14 oz (400 g) can unsweetened chestnut purée
1 teaspoon natural vanilla essence
1 tablespoon walnut or hazelnut oil
1½ pint (300 ml) low-fat yoghurt

Heat the milk to just below boiling point. Whisk together the egg yolks and sugar until pale and fluffy. Add the hot milk, stirring continuously. Return the mixture to the pan and stir over a very low heat until it thickens just enough to coat the back of a spoon. Do not allow the mixture to boil or it will curdle. Leave to cool slightly before stirring in the chestnut purée, vanilla essence and nut oil.

Refrigerate until cool, then stir in the yoghurt. Beat the egg whites until they form stiff peaks and carefully fold into the ice-cream mixture. Pour into a deep container and freeze for 3–4 hours or until firm. This recipe may also be made in an ice cream maker and the mixture should be frozen in the machine according to the manufacturer's instructions. Remove from the freezer about 10 minutes before serving to allow the ice cream to soften slightly.

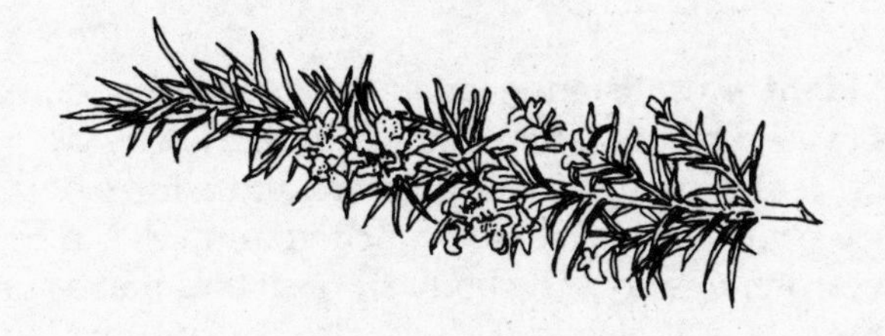

Glossary

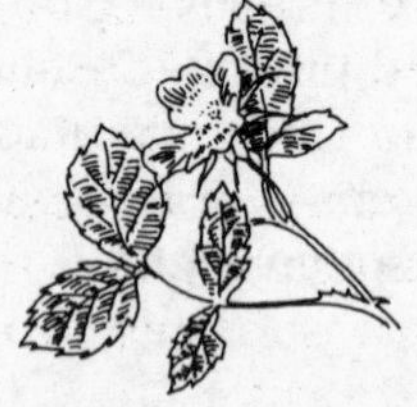

anti-oxidant – a substance capable of preventing damage to cells caused by oxidation and free radical activity.

beta carotene – orange plant pigment and a form of vitamin A (see page 108). While too much vitamin A can be toxic, beta carotene is not. The body stores it and makes vitamin A from it as it needs it. It is also an anti-oxidant (see above).

cell membrane – a double layer of fatty material and proteins that surrounds every living cell.

cholesterol – a fat-like substance produced by the liver and also found in high-fat animal produce. Cholesterol surrounds every cell in the body and is needed to maintain nerve fibres, produce hormones and assist with vitamin D synthesis. The body makes all the cholesterol it needs for these functions. An excess of cholesterol may be deposited in the arteries.

DHA – docosahexaenoic acid. A long-chain Omega-3 polyunsaturated fatty acid found almost exclusively in fish.

EPA – eicosapentaenoic acid. A long-chain Omega-3 polyunsaturated fatty acid found almost exclusively in fish.

essential fatty acids – polyunsaturated fatty acids which are termed 'essential' as they are required for good health. They cannot be synthesized by the body and must be supplied in the diet.

essential oil – fragrant, volatile and highly concentrated essences extracted from leaves, flowers and roots of plants. In this case, 'essential' refers only to the fact that they are essences. They are not for internal use.

free radicals – highly active and destructive chemical compounds produced by oxidation. They are created when a molecular fragment with a single or unpaired electron 'steals' electrons from other molecules.

GLA – gamma-linolenic-acid. A fatty acid occurring naturally in human breast milk, borage oil and evening primrose oil. It can also be produced in the body from linoleic acid.

hydrogenation – the process of combining polyunsaturated oils with hydrogen to convert them into solid fat.

lecithin – a nutritional substance containing fatty acids which is part of the structure of cell membranes.

leukotrienes – biological regulators involved in inflammation in the body.

molecule – two or more atoms held together by pairs of electrons.

monounsaturates – fatty acids containing one double-bond. These are highly resistant to oxidation and are relatively stable at high temperatures. They also have a slight lowering effect on cholesterol in the bloodstream. Examples are olive oil and sesame seed oil.

oxidation – a process whereby a substance is chemically combined with oxygen and its original structure altered or destroyed.

polyunsaturates – fats containing two or more double-bonds. These reduce the level of cholesterol in the bloodstream, but high levels may also adversely affect the balance of other blood fats. Basically, there are two forms of polyunsaturates that end up in our foods. Both *cis* and *trans* fatty acids have equal numbers of carbon atoms and double bonds, but while the cis form is needed by the body to perform many millions of important biological processes, the trans form destabilises cellular activity and undermines good health.

prostaglandins – biological regulators that control many functions in the body.

saturated fats – fatty acids that raise cholesterol levels, usually of animal origin, e.g. butter and lard. Saturated fats also block the health-giving properties of the essential fatty acids.

triglycerides – a molecule of fat or oil consisting of three fatty acid molecules attached to glycerol. This is the form in which fatty acids are stored in the body's fat tissues and in the seeds of plants.

Useful Addresses

Aromatherapy

The International Federation of Aromatherapists
4 Eastmearn Road, London SE21 8HA
Send an SAE for a list of local accredited practitioners and aromatherapy courses. They also publish a regular newsletter which gives details of suppliers of high quality of essential oils.

Aromatherapy Associates
68 The Maltings, Fulmead Street, London SW6
Supply excellent ready-made massage oil blends, electric oil burners and provide occasional training seminars for beauty therapists.

The Association of Tisserand Aromatherapists
PO Box 746, Hove BN3 3XA
Will provide details of aromatherapy training under the direction of Robert Tisserand.

London School of Aromatherapy
PO Box 780, London NW5 1DY
Send a large SAE for details of training courses and a list of their trained aromatherapists country-wide.

Health

The Evening Primrose Office
4 Cupar Road, London SW11 4JW
Offers free help and guidance to the public.

The Institute of Optimum Nutrition
5 Jerdan Place, London SW6
Provides nutritional counselling, seminars and nutrition diploma courses.

National Eczema Society

Tavistock House North, Tavistock Square, London WC1H 9RS

The Arthritis and Rheumatism Council
Copeman House, St Mary's Court, St Mary's Gate, Chesterfield, Derbyshire S41 7TD

ME Action Campaign
PO Box 1302, Wells, BA5 2WE
Will provide information on diet and supplements for this disorder.

Please send an SAE when contacting the above organisations.

General index

Index of recipes

Further Reading

Vital Oils by Liz Earle, Vermilion
The Eskimo Diet by Dr Reg Saynor and Dr Frank Ryan, Ebury Press
Fats, Nutrition and Health by Robert Erdmann Ph.D and Meirion Jones, Thorsons
Evening Primrose Oil by Judy Graham, Thorsons
World of Herbs by Lesley Bremness, Ebury Press
Massage Cures by Nigel Dawes and Fiona Harrold, Thorsons
Smile Therapy by Liz Hodgkinson, Optima
The Sun and Your Skin by Professor Ronald Marks, Optima
Optimum Nutrition by Patrick Holford, ION Press

If you have enjoyed *Save Your Skin with Vital Oils* you may also be interested in *Vital Oils* by Liz Earle, also published by Vermilion. With a wealth of personal and scientific evidence, *Vital Oils* is essential reading for anyone in search of better health and beauty. *Vital Oils* gives an in-depth guide to the special properties of both traditional and newly discovered oils and includes:

- a tried-and-tested two week oil-enriched diet to help you look and feel better
- an at-a-glance guide to oil remedies for health problems
- details on aromatherapy and the therapeutic uses of essential oils
- charts showing the properties of each oil and how it should be used

To obtain your copy, simply complete the coupon below or telephone Merlyn Services on 0279 427203. Your copy will be dispatched to you without delay, postage and packing free.
